AF663866

My research work, with proven track records:

2020*, the result of the clinical trial (by AIIA, Ministry of Ayush) on the DIP diet was released. It is proven to be safe and effective. I introduced the DIP diet in the year 2014. Since then, millions of people could reverse various kind of metabolic disorders including diabetes, high BP, bone disease etc. For the first time the world got effective way to reverse even diabetes type I (as published in the Journal of Science of Healing Outcomes).

2021*, through the observational study conducted by NIN, Ministry of Ayush, my proposed 3-step flu diet was proven to be the only treatment effective to cure even severe COVID (I call it a flu) with zero mortality and zero side effects. Since June 2020 we cured more than 60,000 COVID (flu) patients with Zero Death and Zero Medication.

2022*, the observational study was done to see the effectiveness of my invention, the GRAD system, in reversing kidney failure among dialysis patients. The study concluded that 75% of the dialysis patients could free themselves of the dependency on dialysis. The study was accepted by prestigious 'International Journal of Healthcare Management'.

2023*, I hereby present the "Rabbit – Tortoise model for cancer cure", and through this book the method effective in reversing various kind of cancer and getting rid of all kind of tumors, cysts, fibroids, polyps and other outgrowths. The book comprises the science of my innovation, including evidences from scientific literature, successful testimonials and results of the observational study (conducted in Dayanand Ayurvedic College, Jalandhar), on the effectiveness of the Rabbit-Tortoise Model.

***Go to the following link, to access the clinical trials/observational studies.** www.biswaroop.com/research-papers

Rabbit-Tortoise Model for CANCER CURE

Dr. Biswaroop Roy Chowdhury

India Office:
C/o India Book of Records
B-121, 2nd Floor, Greenfields,
Faridabad -120003 (Haryana),
India
Ph.: +91-9312286540

Malaysia Office:
C/o Bishwaroop International Healing & Research
PT 573, Lot 15077 Jalan Tuanku
Munawir,
70000 Negeri Sembilan, Malaysia
Tel: +6012-2116089

Vietnam Office:
C/o Vietnam Book of Records
148 Hong Ha Street
9 Award, Phu Nhuan District,
Ho Chi Minh City, Vietnam
- Hotline: (+84) 903710505

Switzerland Office:
C/o Nigel Kingsley
Kraftwerkstr. 95, ch-5465, Mellikon,
Switzerland
Tel: 0041 79 222 2323

FOLLOW ME

Facebook: https://www.facebook.com/drbrc.official/
Twitter: https://twitter.com/drbiswarooproy
Bitchute: https://www.bitchute.com/channel/drbiswarooproychowdhury/
Instagram: https://www.instagram.com/dr.biswarooproychowdhury/
Telegram: https://t.me/drbiswarooproychowdhury
Email: biswaroop@biswaroop.com
Website: www.biswaroop.com
Video Channel: www.coronakaal.tv

Research : Rachna Sharma
Graphics Designer: Shankar Singh Koranga
Video Translation: Shilpa Tiwari
Proof Reading: Raj Kishore Gupta
Compilation: Shruti Vatsa
Testimonial collection: Dr. Sanju Khari

Published by
Dynamic Memory Pvt. Ltd.
B-121, 2nd Floor, Greenfields, Faridabad- 121003 (Haryana)
Mob: +91-9312286540 email: biswaroop@biswaroop.com
website: www.biswaroop.com

Dedication

Dedicated to my angel daughter Ivy,

loving wife Neerja

&

caring parents

Shri Bikash Roy Chowdhury

Shrimati Lila Roy Chowdhury

CONTENTS

CHAPTER -1

The Rabbit – Tortoise Model

The word "Cancer" for most of the people, even the doctors, means suffering and death! But not for my patients. Hundreds of my patients including those who got themselves admitted in any of my HIIMS hospitals or got in touch with me through Virtual OPD, are free of fear and are able to get out of the trap of cancer. Now with the goal to reach more and more people, especially those, who are suffering and unable to reach me, I present the "Rabbit-Tortoise Model for Cancer Cure". Just by following the four rules of this method, one can empower himself with a strategy to heal.

In the Rabbit-Tortoise model, 'tortoise' represents an 'indolent cancer cell', which sits silently in your body life-long without harming you and the 'rabbit' represents the 'aggressive cancer cells', which jump from one organ to other and has a potential to harm.

The four rules of Rabbit-Tortoise model are as follows:

Rule 1: Each one of us have detectable indolent 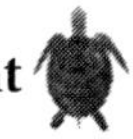 cancer cells.

99.9% [1] of the circulating tumour in our body never matures to form a secondary growth. Upon autopsy of thyroid, prostate and breast, and of the people who died with causes other than cancer, 100% of the thyroid specimen, 70% of prostate and 40% of breast specimen were found to be cancerous[2].

This means, had the individuals gone for a voluntary cancer diagnosis when alive, most of them would have been declared as cancer patients followed by lethal and unnecessary chemotherapy, radiation or surgery. Such indolent cancer cells, which are often also known as pseudocancer[2] or incidentalomas [2], are also found frequently in other body organs including lungs and blood as well. Often it is presumed and widely believed that a cancer cell will progress from stage I to stage IV and finally will cause death[3].

Linear model of cancer progression

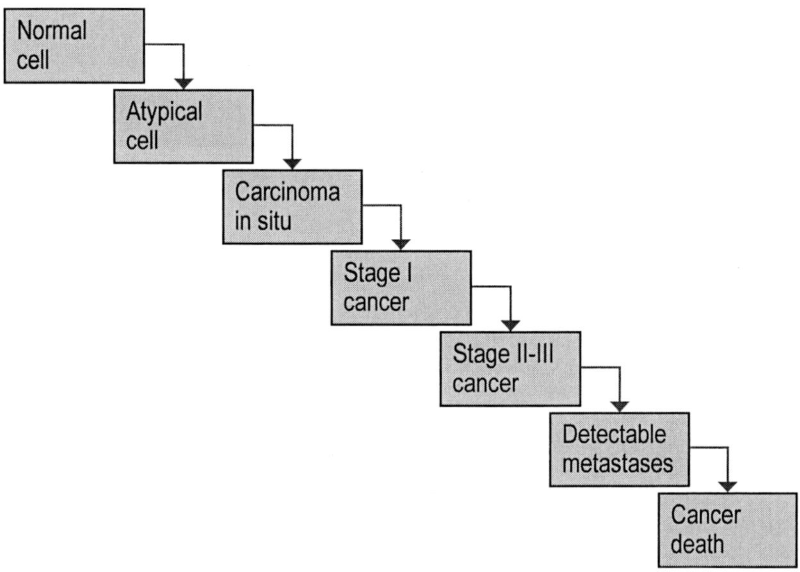

Whereas the truth is that an aggressively growing tumour regresses on its own (as shown on page no. 11) and settles down as an indolent cancer cell for the rest of the life without causing any harm[3].

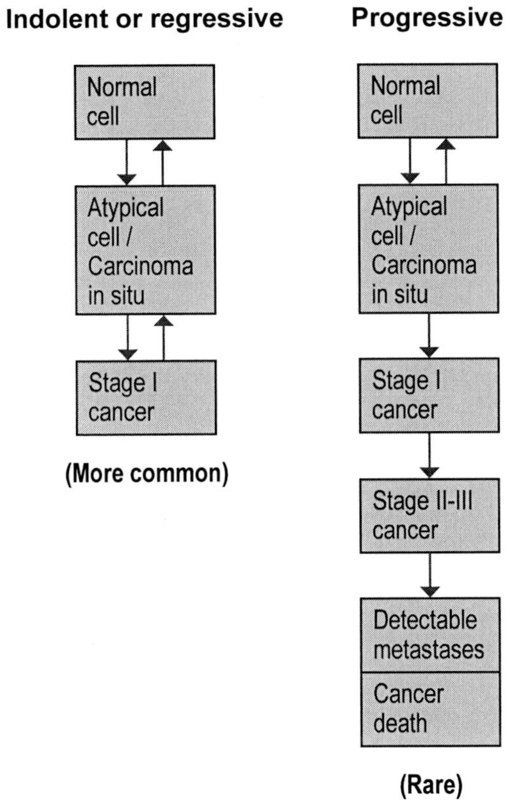

This phenomenon is often known as disease reservoir[4], this means - potentially harmful looking cancer cells (harmful from the point of view of a pathologist/radiologist) never cause any harm[2]. With the above understanding that most of the cancer cells are harmless and, in many instances, even the aggressive cancer cells often regress on their own, the safe method to know whether cancer cells in the body are causing life-threatening damage or not, the best way is to track the haemoglobin level. You will find more on tracking haemoglobin level to diagnose truly life-threatening cancer in chapter 2, whereas why we should avoid biopsy/mammogram etc, you will find in rule 2.

Rule 2: Biopsy (or any other diagnostic test) cannot distinguish between indolent & aggressive cancer.

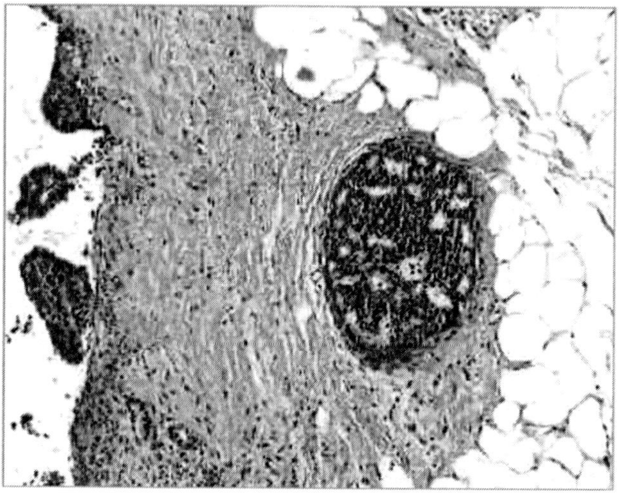

The above biopsy sample was shown to trained pathologists from eight US states, with an objective to estimate the magnitude of disagreements among the pathologist. 33%, 48% & 19% of the pathologists diagnosed the biopsy slide as normal, abnormal and cancerous respectively.[4] This disagreement points out a serious flaw in the science of biopsy which otherwise is known to be the gold standard of cancer diagnosis. It also means that the fate of the patient's treatment depends on a diagnostic method which is no more accurate than a coin toss. This ambiguity was clearly demonstrated in a study[4] on pathologists where among the biopsy slides of abnormal cells, 52% of the pathologists' interpretation was not in accordance to the consensus derived reference. The reason for this interpretation failure can be understood with the help of 'Soil and Seed' hypothesis proposed by an English surgeon Steven Paget in 1889[5].

In this model, seed represents the cancer cell. The seed even though has a great and undeniable potential to grow, it will grow or not - always depends on the potency of the soil, in this case the soil represents the surrounding of the cancer cells. The most fertile ground for the cancer cells to grow is when the surrounding has chemical changes similar to that of a wound healing process[6].

The flow chart given below represents the mechanism of wound healing:

Normal Wound Healing and Tumor Growth

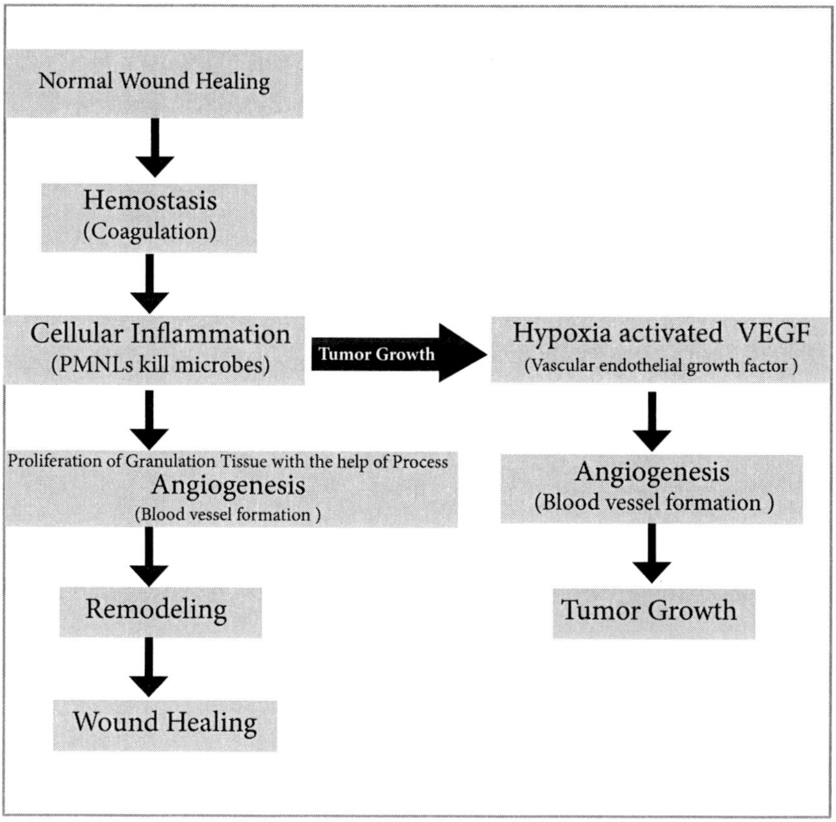

Similar is the mechanism of surrounding the cancer cells in its proliferation with only one exception i.e., the mechanism of wound healing process carries on endlessly to unusual growth[6].

The above explanation makes it clear that there is a very thin line of difference between the indolent and aggressive cancer cells and these are not distinguishable with the modern widespread diagnostics like biopsy or PET scan. As a result of it often the following non-lethal cells are misinterpreted as cancer [7] :

1. Nipple adenoma
2. Syringomatous tumour of nipple
3. Radical scar
4. Sclerosing adenosis
5. Micro glandular adenosis
6. Intraduct papilloma
7. Fibroadenoma
8. Pleomorphic adenoma
9. Benign spindle cell lesion
10. Scar tissues
11. Fibromatosis
12. Nodular fasciitis
13. Pseudo angiomatous stromal hyperplasia
14. Myofibroblastoma
15. Histiocytic inflammation
16. Granular cell tumour

Besides the danger of misinterpretation of the above benign condition as cancer, the biopsy often leads to epithelial cell displacement following needling procedure leading to subsequent excision specimens misdiagnosed as cancer. [8]

It is well established that the biopsies suppress the immune system and promote cancer metastasis. [9, 10, 11, 12, 13]

The above evidence proves the worthlessness of biopsy. However, the equally alarming aspect of biopsy is the immediate damage it causes to the patients which includes moderate to heavy bleeding, unbearable pain, brain damage and even death.

Immediate Complications of Biopsy [14]	
1. Pain	84% [15]
2. Severe Bleeding	0.16%[16,17,18,19,20,21,22]
3. Infection	13.5%[23]
4. Puncture of Viscera	0.1%[24,25]
5. Death	0.11%[26,27,28,23,29,30,24]
6. Tumour Recurrence	Significantly High[31]
7. Colon Puncture	0.033%[32]
8. Kidney Puncture	0.033%[32]
9. Gallbladder Puncture	0.013%[32]

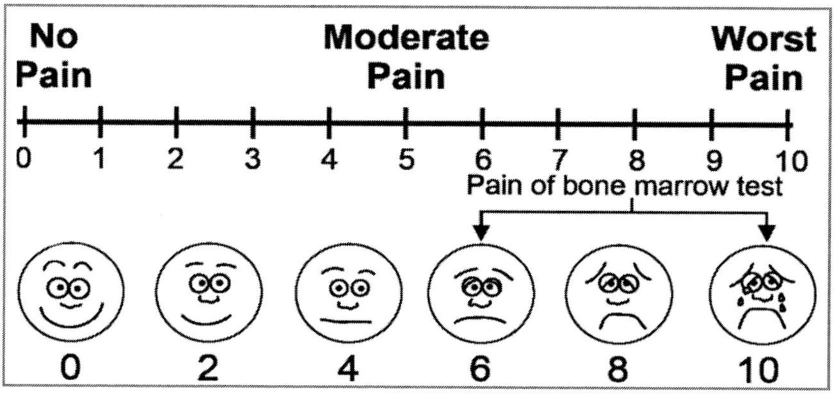

Pain Scale

Similarly, in the case of mammography, the breast is tightly and often painfully[30] compressed between two imaging plates. The cumulative effect of routine mammography screening may increase women's risk of developing radiation-induced breast cancer [33] and if cancer is present in the breast, the compression can result in metastasis[34].

On the contrary, avoiding repeated mammography may lead to at least 22% chances of spontaneous regression.

In other words, by simply avoiding the repeated dose of ionizing radiation administered during mammography, the body is given a chance to heal on its own and often it does[35].

In fact, cancer diagnostics is the fuel behind the cancerous growth of the cancer industry. For further reading on cancer diagnostics read chapter 3, 'How to Invent a Cancer' patent?'

Radiation / Chemotherapy

Rule 3: Indolent 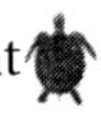 Cancer ⟶ Aggressive 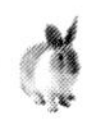 Cancer

Biopsy/Surgery

To start with, we have to recognize, more and more healthy people are labelled as cancer patients and this is achieved by cancer industry by:

1. **Changing the definition of cancer itself:** Biopsy once defined as a normal might now be defined as stage1 cancer.[36,37] The terms like precancerous and premalignant are introduced resulting in more people becoming eligible for cancer treatment.
2. **Large scale unnecessary screening:** Overwhelming increase in screening in last 50 years leading to undoubtedly detecting indolent disease, best exemplified in prostate cancer,[38,39] breast cancer,[40] and even lung cancer.[41, 42, 43] The result of large screening program

(476694 children) in Quebec, Canada, showed that screening was not effective and in fact was harmful.[44]

3. **Applying excessive pressure during mammography:** Mammography involves compressing the breasts between two plates in order to spread out the breast tissue for imaging. Today's mammogram equipment applies 19 kg of pressure to the breasts. Not surprisingly, this can cause significant pain. However, there is also a serious health risk associated with the compression applied to the breasts. Only 10 kg of pressure is needed to rupture the encapsulation of a cancerous tumor.[45] The amount of pressure involved in a mammography procedure therefore has the potential to rupture existing tumours and spread malignant cells into the bloodstream.[46]

Recent evidence shows that cutting out a tumour either provides no benefit to the patients[47, 48] or increases the mortality.[49, 50, 51]

The more the body is cut, the worse is the outcome.

Cancer metastasis is the primary cause of most cancer deaths[52, 53, 54] and yes, the public remains unaware that surgical removal of tumour causes cancer metastasis.[55, 56, 57, 58, 59, 60, 61, 62]

Similarly laparotomy or mastectomy could promote tumour growth and angiogenesis in ovarian cancer.[63]

Removal of the primary colorectal cancer correlated with increased risk of liver metastasis. Surgery-induced inflammation may facilitate metastasis by altering the distant microenvironment. In a recent paper, it was reported that reactive oxygen species (ROS) were produced by macrophages (Kupffer cells) during surgery, which altered the ultrastructure of the liver and promoted cancer cell adhesion.[64] In clinical practices, removing primary tumours is accompanied by an exceptionally rapid metastatic outgrowth in many cases, which are in line with experimental evidence. For example, Peters et al. showed a marked increase in proliferation and a significant decrease in apoptosis in metastatic lesions,[65] which suggests that metastasis is influenced by surgical resection of primary tumour in human.

Similarly, there are no evidences to prove that chemotherapy helps a cancer patient to improve his quality of life or increase his life span. On the contrary, there are sufficient evidences to prove otherwise.[66, 67, 68, 69]

Here the point to understand is the shrinking of the initial tumour mass; chemotherapy deceives the doctors into thinking that the patients are benefitting from the treatment, when in reality, the growth and spread of cancer gets accelerated by it.

Likewise, there are no evidences to prove that radiotherapy can help a cancer patient improve his quality of life or increase his lifespan. On the contrary, there are sufficient evidences to prove otherwise.[70, 71, 72, 73]

Rule 4: Aggressive 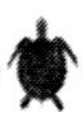 Cancer —Resetting / Body Clock→ Indolent 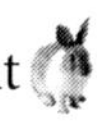 Cancer

Through rule 2, we know in minority of us, rabbit kind of cancer cells are present leading to causing tumorous growth, organ damage, pain/suffering and death. With the evidence in rule-3, now we know that one of the major causes of such progression is chemotherapy, radiation, surgery or even diagnostics like biopsy and mammogram; however, the major cause of formation and progression of rabbit type cancer cell is disruption of your body's circadian clock – circadian clock, the noble prize-winning science - 2017, is the central controller[74] of your health. The deviation and the disruption of the circadian clock led to initiation of not just cancer progression but also causes your body becoming the fertile ground for all kind of illnesses including metabolic syndrome, heart/kidney failure and all kind of outgrowth (polyps, fibroid, cysts, stone etc.).

What is circadian/body clock?

It's all about timing. Let's start with the beginning of the origin of time. The earth makes one rotation on its axis, which leads to day-night 24 hrs cycle, effecting the physiology of all living organisms.

Our inner world, i.e., each and every cell, tissue and the organ itself function in rhythmic manner with one cycle equals to 24 hrs, strictly in coordination with the earth's each rotation around its axis. One of the major gateways which connect, each and every cell of our body to the outer world (Earth's rotation on its axis) is the eye which keeps a tract of light-dark cycle of earth and signals the suprachiasmatic nucleus (SCN), a small brain region containing 10000 – 15000 neurons located in hypothomes. SCN as a master timekeeper (based on the various external signals like light-dark cycle, fast-feed cycle etc), relays signal to the clock protein of each and every cell/organ of the body. SCN as a concert master of an orchestra, directs each and every organ to play the music of life in harmony with each other. Now imagine an orchestra without a concert master or with poorly trained concert master. Even if each of the musician is playing his respective organ at its best but lack of direction will lead to the ultimate outcome as a noise rather than a music. Similarly, it is seen through experiments on mice, surgical removal of SCN or through observational studies[75] on humans, when light-dark cycle and fast-feed cycle are distorted in humans, due to poor lifestyle choices like too much of light at night[76] (LAN) or feeding[77] late night and fasting during day (as often happens among shift workers), the rhythmic coordinating between the organs is lost, leading to manifestation of various illnesses. In fact, in a healthy body, there is a rhythm (24 hrs cycle) in various aspects of functional coordination between the organs. For example,

1. The 24 hrs. Blood Pressure Rhythm:

For most of us the health B.P. cycle can be identified as:

1) Highest B.P. around 10 AM

2) Lowest B.P. around 10 PM

3) The difference between the highest & the lowest being 10 to 20%.[78]

Any deviation from the above may mean disruption of the body's central circadian clock (SCN) leading to progression towards illness.

Any deviation from the above may mean disruption of the body's central circadian clock (SCN) leading to progression towards illness.

2. The 24 hrs body temperature rhythm:

For most of us, the peak body temperature is near 6 pm and the lowest body temperature is near 6 am, [79] with average temperature > 37^{0}C and the difference between the lowest and highest always less than 0.6^{0}C.[80] Deviation from the above may mean, your progression towards illness.

3. The circadian clock of urine output:

The urine production during the time you are awake is expected to be at least 3 times the urine production during the night sleep time.[78] Deviation from it may hint impaired kidney functioning.

4. Pancreas are known to work best at around 8 am and work the least at or after 8 pm: [81]

Feeding yourself away from this time bracket (8 am to 8 pm) may mean disruption of central circadian clock leading to hosting illness.

5. Circadian rhythm of sleep-wake up cycle:

Major melatonin production at a night and major cortisol production since morning leads to sleep at night and alertness during the day.[82] Any deviation from it may cause insomnia, depression, low immunity, poor mental functioning etc.

Various clock gene, a kind of protein located in each and every cell of our body, as a timekeeper work in coordination with SCN, it maintains the above 24 hrs rhythm of various inter/intra organ functioning & leading to maintenance of health and the life itself.

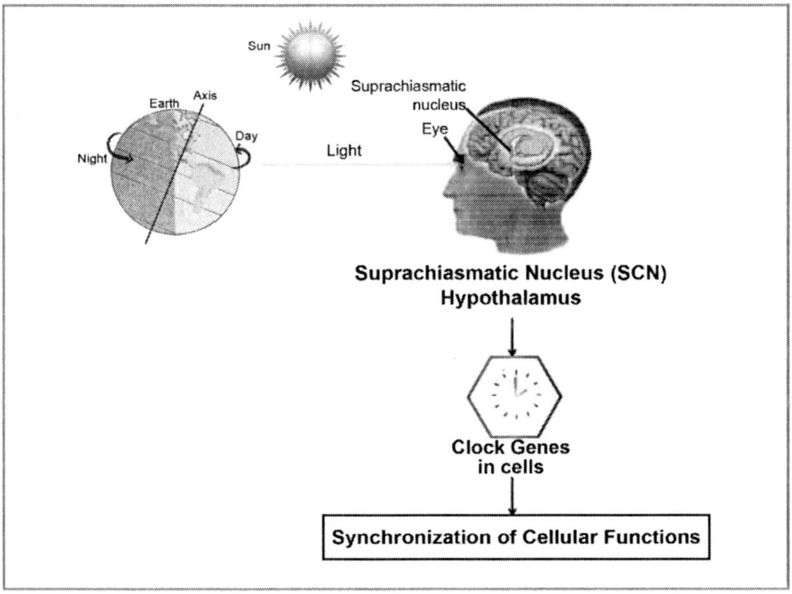

While the clock genes in cells maintain the intrinsic timing keeping in sync with the external environment via SCN mediated through the eye, leading to SCN mediated through the eye, leading to maintain the balance of 24 hrs cycle of blood pressure, core body temperature, urine output, sleep wake up hormone secretion, high low cycle of insulin production among other aspects of 24 hrs cycle.

In the industrial world, this flow of information (as shown in the previous diagram) is interrupted in many ways. One of them being light at night (LAN)[76] leading to disruption in the production of melatonin / oestrogen causing chronic inflammation and lowering production of killer cells resulting in DNA damage, making a ground for cancer proliferation.

Meta analysis[76] of studies on the impact of LAN on shift workers and flight attendants concluded increase in the chances of breast / prostate / rectal cancer among others, sometime as high as 5 times.[75]

Similarly expanding the time window of eating beyond the peak functioning of pancreas (8 am to 8 pm) also correlates to increase in death due to cancer. [83]

Interestingly it has been observed through various observational studies on humans and clinical trials on mice by correcting the circadian clock one cannot only halt the progression of cancer (and most of the lifestyle-oriented diseases) but also disease can be reversed. [84., 82]

Following factors are proven to be helpful in correction of the circadian clock:

1) Limiting the light exposure after sunset.[85]
2) Limiting the feeding time within the window of 10 hrs (between 8 am to 6 pm). [86]
3) Grounding the body every day. [87]
4) Calorie-light food with dietary phyto-chemicals as a major part of the diet. [88]
5) Core body temperature fall is a part of therapy to induce restful sleep.[89, 90]

Ahead in the book the chapters - Resetting the Body Clock & Circadian Dining Table - will give more insight on the mechanism reversing illness by correcting circadian clock.

References:

1. *Akhtar, Mohammed MD,; Haider, Abdulrazzaq MD*; Rashid, Sameera MD†; Al-Nabet, Ajayeb Dakhilalla M.H. Paget's "Seed and Soil" Theory of Cancer Metastasis: An Idea Whose Time has Come. Advances In Anatomic Pathology 26(1):p 69-74, January 2019.*

2. *H. Gilbert Welch, William C. Black, Overdiagnosis in Cancer, JNCI: Journal of the National Cancer Institute, Volume 102, Issue 9, 5 May 2010, Pages 605–613*

3. *Esserman LJ, Thompson IM, Reid B, Nelson P, Ransohoff DF, Welch HG, Hwang S, Berry DA, Kinzler KW, Black WC, Bissell M, Parnes H, Srivastava S. Addressing overdiagnosis and overtreatment in cancer: a prescription for change. Lancet Oncol. 2014 May;15(6):e234-42. doi: 10.1016/S1470-2045(13)70598-9. PMID: 24807866; PMCID: PMC4322920.*

4. *Elmore JG, Longton GM, Carney PA, Geller BM, Onega T, Tosteson AN, Nelson HD, Pepe MS, Allison KH, Schnitt SJ, O'Malley FP, Weaver DL. Diagnostic concordance among pathologists interpreting breast biopsy specimens. JAMA. 2015 Mar 17;313(11):1122-32. doi: 10.1001/jama.2015.1405. PMID: 25781441; PMCID: PMC4516388.*

5. *Liu, Q., Zhang, H., Jiang, X. et al. Factors involved in cancer metastasis: a better understanding to "seed and soil" hypothesis. Mol Cancer 16, 176 (2017). https://doi.org/10.1186/s12943-017-0742-4.*

6. *Dvorak HF. Tumors: wounds that do not heal-redux. Cancer Immunol Res. 2015 Jan;3(1):1-11. doi: 10.1158/2326-6066.CIR-14-0209. PMID: 25568067; PMCID: PMC4288010.*

7. *Quinn, C., Maguire, A. and Rakha, E. (2023), Pitfalls in breast pathology. Histopathology, 82: 140-161. https://doi.org/10.1111/his.14799*

8. *Youngson BJ, Cranor M, Rosen PP. Epithelial displacement in surgical breast specimens following needling procedures. Am. J. Surg. Pathol. 1994; 18; 896–903.*

9. *Hobson J, Gummadidala P, Silverstrim B, et al. Acute inflammation induced by the biopsy of mouse mammary tumors promotes the development of metastasis. Breast Cancer Res Treat. 2013; 139(2):391-401.*

10. *Miller AB, To T, Baines CJ, Wall C. Canadian National Breast Screening Study-2: 13-year results of a randomized trial in women aged 50-59 years. J Natl Cancer Inst. 2000; 92(18):1490-9. 46*

11. *Kornguth PJ, Keefe FJ, Conaway MR. Pain during mammography: characteristics and relationship to demographic and medical variables. Pain. 1996; 66(2-3):187-94.*

12. *Van netten JP, Cann SA, Hall JG. Mammography controversies: time for informed consent? J Natl Cancer Inst. 1997; 89(15):1164-5.*

13. *Zahl PH, Maehlen J, Welch HG. The natural history of invasive breast cancers detected by screening mammography. Arch Intern Med. 2008; 168 (21):2311-6.*

14. *Complications of Liver Biopsy - Risk Factors, Management and Recommendations written by Norman O neil Machado Submitted: November 28th, 2010 Published: September 6th, 2011 DOI: 10.5772/23600.*

15. *Eisenberg E. Konopniki M. Veitsman E. Kramskay R. Gaintini D. Baruch Y. 2003 Prevalence and characteristics of pain induced by percutaneous liver biopsy. Anaesth Analg.;96 5 1392 96.*

16. *Ghent CN. 2006 Percutaneous liver biopsy : Reflections and refinements. Can J Gastroenterol.;20 2 75 9.*

17. *Rockey DC, Caldwell SH, Goodman ZD, Nelson RC, Smith AD. 2009 Liver biopsy. Hepatology.;49 3 1017 1044.*

18. *Siegel CA, Silas AW, Suriawinata AA, van Leeuwen DJ. Liver biopsy 2005 When and how ? Cleve Clin J Med.;72 3 199 224.*

19. *Friedman LS. 2004Controversies in liver biopsy: who, where, when, how, why?. Curr Gastroenterol Rep.;6 1 30 36.*

20. *Minuk GY, Sutherland LR, Wiseman DA, MacDonald FR, Ding DL. 1987 Prospective study of the incidence of ultrasound detected intrahepatic and subcapsular haematoma in patients randomized to 6 or 24 hours of bed rest after percutaneous liver biopsy. Gastroenetrology.;92 2 290 93.*

21. *Lankisch P. G. Thiele E. Mahlke R. Lubbers H. Riesner K. 1990 Prospective study of the incidence of ultrasound detected hepatic haematomas 2 to 24 hours after percutaneous liver biopsy. Z Gastroenterol.;28 5 247 50.*

22. *Sugano S. Sumino Y. Hatori T. Mizugami H. Kuwafuni T. Abei T. 1991Incidence of ultrasound detected intrahepatic haematoma due to trucut needle liver biopsy. Dig Dis Sci.;36 9 1229 33.*

23. *Piccinino F. Sagnelli E. Pasquale G. Giusti G. 1986 Complications following percutaneous liver biopsy. A multicentre retrospective study on 68,276 biopsies. J Hepatol.;2 1 165 73.*

24. *Lublin M. Danforth D. N. 2001 Iatrogenic gall bladder perforation: conservative management by percutaneous drainage and cholecystectomy. Am Surg.;67 8 760 63.*

25. *Ahluwalia JP, LaBrecque DR. 2004A large bilioma causing gastric outlet obstruction after a percutaneous liver biopsy. J Clin Gastroenterol.;38 6 535 39.*

26. *Mc Gill D. B. Rakela J. Zinsmeister A. R. Ott B. J. 1990A 21 year experience with major haemorrhage after percutaneous liver biopsy. Gastroenterology.;99 5 1396 1400.*

27. *Riley TR 3rd. 1999 How often does ultrasound marking change the liver biopsy site ? Am J Gastroenetrol.;94 11 3320 22.*

28. *Tan K. T. Rajan D. K. Kachura J. R. Hayeems E. ME Simons Ho. C. S. 2005 Pain after percutaneous liver biopsy for diffuse hepatic disease: a randomized trial comparing subcostal and intercostal approaches. J Vas Interv Radiol.;16 9 1215 19.*

29. *DiMichele DM, Hathaway WE. 1990 Use of DDAVP in inherited and acquired platelet dysfunction. Am J Haematol.;33 1 39 45.*

30. *Bubak ME, Porayko MK, Krom RA, Wiesner RH, 1991 Complications of liver biopsy in liver transplant patients: increased sepsis associated with choledochojejunostomy. Hepatology.:14(6);1063 1065.*

31. *Relevance of Compartmental Anatomic Guidelines for Biopsy of Musculoskeletal Tumors: Retrospective Review of 363 Biopsies over a 6-Year Period UyBico, Stacy J. et al.Journal of Vascular and Interventional Radiology, Volume 23, Issue 4, 511 - 518.e2.*

32. *Complications following percutaneous liver biopsy. A multicentre Retrospective Study on 68276 Biopsies. Piccinino, F. et al. Journal of Hepatology, Volume 2, Issue 2, 165 - 173.*

33. *Miglioretti DL, Lange J, van den Broek JJ, Lee CI, van Ravesteyn NT, Ritley D, Kerlikowske K, Fenton JJ, Melnikow J, de Koning HJ, Hubbard RA. Radiation-Induced Breast Cancer Incidence and Mortality from Digital Mammography Screening: A Modeling Study. Ann Intern Med. 2016 Feb 16;164(4):205-14. doi: 10.7326/M15-1241. Epub 2016 Jan 12. PMID: 26756460; PMCID: PMC4878445.*

34. *Relevance of Compartmental Anatomic Guidelines for Biopsy of Musculoskeletal Tumors: Retrospective Review of 363 Biopsies over a 6-Year Period UyBico, Stacy J. et al. Journal of Vascular and Interventional Radiology, Volume 23, Issue 4, 511 - 518.e2.*

35. *Complications following percutaneous liver biopsy. A multicentre Retrospective Study on 68276 Biopsies. Piccinino, F. et al.Journal of Hepatology, Volume 2, Issue 2, 165 - 173.*

36. *Welch HG, Woloshin S, Schwartz LM. Skin biopsy rates and incidence of melanoma: population based ecological study. BMJ. 2005;331:481.*

37. *Levell NJ, Beattie CC, Shuster S, Greenberg DC. Melanoma epidemic: a midsummer night's dream? Br J Dermatol. 2009;161:630–34*

38. *Wilt TJ, Brawer MK, Jones KM, et al. Radical prostatectomy versus observation for localized prostate cancer. N Engl J Med. 2012;367:203–13.*

39. *Thompson IM, Jr, Tangen CM. Prostate cancer—uncertainty and a way forward. N Engl J Med. 2012;367:270–71.*

40. *Esserman L, Shieh Y, Thompson I. Rethinking screening for breast cancer and prostate cancer. JAMA. 2009;302:1685–92.*

41. *Bach PB, Jett JR, Pastorino U, Tockman MS, Swensen SJ, Begg CB. Computed tomography screening and lung cancer outcomes. JAMA. 2007;297:953–61.*

42. *Bach PB. Is our natural-history model of lung cancer wrong? Lancet Oncol. 2008;9:693–97.*

43. *Humphrey LL, Deffebach M, Pappas M, et al. Screening for lung cancer with low-dose computed tomography: a systematic review to update the US Preventive services task force recommendation. Ann Intern Med. 2013;159:411–20.*

44. *Woods WG, Gao RN, Shuster JJ, et al. Screening of infants and mortality due to neuroblastoma. N Engl J Med. 2002;346:1041–46.*

45. *The Downside of Mammograms - Kresser Institute.*

46. *Sahar, S., Sassone-Corsi, P. Metabolism and cancer: the circadian clock connection. Nat Rev Cancer 9, 886–896 (2009). https://doi.org/10.1038/nrc2747.*

47. *Shalowitz DI, Epstein AJ, Buckingham L, Ko EM, Giuntoli RL. Survival implications of time to surgical treatment of endometrial cancers. Am J Obstet Gynecol. 2016.*

48. *Bethune R, Sbaih M, Brosnan C, Arulampalam T. What happens when we do not operate? Survival following conservative bowel cancer management. Ann R Coll Surg Engl. 2016; 98(6):409-12.*

49. *Langley RR, Fidler IJ. Tumor cell-organ microenvironment interactions in the pathogenesis of cancer metastasis. Endocr Rev. 2007; 28(3):297-321. 50.*

50. *Langley RR, Fidler IJ. The seed and soil hypothesis revisited–the role of tumor stroma interactions in metastasis to different organs. Int J Cancer. 2011; 128(11):2527-35.*

5. *Chen LL, Blumm N, Christakis NA, Barabási AL, Deisboeck TS. Cancer metastasis networks and the prediction of progression patterns. Br J Cancer. 2009; 101(5):749-58.*

52. *Cole WH. Spontaneous regression of cancer: the metabolic triumph of the host? Ann N Y Acad Sci. 1974; 230:111-41.*

53. *Lange PH, Hekmat K, Bos! G, Kennedy BJ, Fraley EE. Acclerated growth of testicular cancer after cytoreductive surgery. Cancer. 1980; 45(6):1498-506.*

54. *Demicheli R, Retsky MW, Hrushesky WJ, Baum M. Tumor dormancy and surgery driven interruption of dormancy in breast cancer: learning from failures. Nat Clin Pract Oncol. 2007; 4(12):699-710.*

55. *Retsky MW, Demicheli R, Hrushesky WJ, Baum M, Gukas ID. Dormancy and surgery driven escape from dormancy help explain some clinical features of breast cancer. APMIS. 2008; 116(7-8):730-41.*

56. *Goldstein MR, Mascitelli L. Surgery and cancer promotion: are we trading beauty for cancer? QJM. 2011; 104(9):811-5.*

57. *Hanin L, Bunimovich-mendrazitsky S. Reconstruction of the natural history of metastatic cancer and assessment of the effects of surgery: Gompertzian growth of the primary tumor. Math Biosci.2014; 247:4758.51.*

58. *Hanin L, Pavlova L. A quantitative insight into metastatic relapse of breast cancer. J Theor Biol. 2016; 394:172-81.*

59. *Sano F, Ueda K, Murakami J, Hayashi M, Nishimoto A, Hamano K. Enhanced tumor growth in the remaining lung after major lung resection. J Surg Res. 2016; 202(1):1-7.*

60. *Effects of radiotherapy and surgery in early breast cancer. An overview of the randomized trials. Early Breast Cancer Trialists' Collaborative Group. N Engl J Med. 1995; 333(22):1444-55.*

61. *Adjuvant radiotherapy for rectal cancer: a systematic overview of 8,507 patients from 22 randomised trials. Lancet. 2001; 358(9290):1291-304.*

62. *Clarke M, Collins R, Darby S, et al. Effects of radiotherapy and of differences in the extent of surgery for early breast cancer on local recurrence and 15-year survival: an overview of the randomized trials. Lancet. 2005; 366(9503):2087-106.*

63. *Lee JW, Shahzad MM, Lin YG, Armaiz-Pena G, Mangala LS, Han HD, Kim HS, Nam EJ, Jennings NB, Halder J et al.: Surgical stress promotes tumor growth in ovarian carcinoma. Clin Cancer Res 2009, 15(8):Clin Cancer Res–2702.*

64. *Gul N, Bogels M, Grewal S, van der Meer AJ, Rojas LB, Fluitsma DM, van den Tol MP, Hoeben KA, van Marle J, de Vries HE, et al. Surgery-induced reactive oxygen species enhance colon carcinoma cell binding by disrupting the liver endothelial cell lining. Gut. 2011;60(8):1076–86.*

65. *Peeters CF, de Waal RM, Wobbes T, Westphal JR, Ruers TJ. Outgrowth of human liver metastases after resection of the primary colorectal tumor: a shift in the balance between apoptosis and proliferation. Int J Cancer. 2006;119(6):1249–53.*

66. *Owusu C, Margevicius S, Schlucter M, Koroukian SM, Schmitz KH,Berger NA. Vulnerable elders survey and socioeconomic status predict functional decline and death among older women with newly diagnosed non metastatic breast cancer. Cancer 2016; 122 (16): 2579-86.*

67. *Dao, T. L. and Kovaric, J.: Incidence of Pulmonary and Skin Metastases in Women with Breast Cancer Who Received Postoperative Irradiation. Surgery, 52:203, 1962.*

68. *DeCourmelles, F.: Action Atrophique Glandulaire Des Rayons X. C. R. Acad. Sci (Paris), 140:606, 1905.*

69. *Fisher B, Slack NH, Cavanaugh PJ, Gardner B, Ravdin RG. Postoperative radiotherapy in the treatment of breast cancer: results of the NSABP clinical trial. Ann Surg. 1970; 172(4):711-32.49.*

70. *Stjernswärd J. Decreased survival related to irradiation postoperatively in early operable breast cancer. Lancet. 1974; 2(7892):1285-6./4(16,18), 2/4 (17,143,144), 2/5 (20-22) , 2/5 (25),2/7 (28-34).*

71. *Wilt TJ, Brawer MK, Jones KM, et al. Radical prostatectomy versus observation for localized prostate cancer. N Engl J Med. 2012;367(3):203-13.*

72. *Vila J, Gandini S, Gentilini 0. Overall survival according to type of surgery in young (<40 years) early breast cancer patients: A systematic meta-analysis comparing breast-conserving surgery versus mastectomy. Breast. 2015; 24(3):175-81.*

73. *Jacobson JA, Danforth DN, Cowan KH, et al. Ten-year results of a comparison of Engl J Med. 1995; 332(14):907-11.*

74. *Sahar, S., Sassone-Corsi, P. Metabolism and cancer: the circadian clock connection. Nat Rev Cancer 9, 886–896 (2009). https://doi.org/10.1038/nrc2747*

75. *Sulli G, Lam MTY, Panda S. Interplay between Circadian Clock and Cancer: New Frontiers for Cancer Treatment. Trends Cancer. 2019 Aug;5(8):475-494. doi: 10.1016/j.trecan.2019.07.002.*

76. *Urbano T, Vinceti M, Wise LA, Filippini T. Light at night and risk of breast cancer: a systematic review and dose-response meta-analysis. Int J Health Geogr. 2021 Oct 16;20(1):44. doi: 10.1186/s12942-021-00297-7. PMID: 34656111; PMCID: PMC8520294.*

77. *Filipski E, Innominato PF, Wu M, Li XM, Iacobelli S, Xian LJ, Lévi F. Effects of light and food schedules on liver and tumor molecular clocks in mice. J Natl Cancer Inst. 2005 Apr 6;97(7):507-17. doi: 10.1093/jnci/dji083. Erratum in: J Natl Cancer Inst. 2005 May 18;97(10):780. PMID: 15812076.*

78. *Stow LR, Gumz ML. The circadian clock in the kidney. J Am Soc Nephrol. 2011 Apr;22(4):598-604. doi: 10.1681/ASN.2010080803. Epub 2011 Mar 24. PMID: 21436284; PMCID: PMC5797999.*

79. *Harding EC, Franks NP, Wisden W. The Temperature Dependence of Sleep. Front Neurosci. 2019 Apr 24;13:336. doi: 10.3389/fnins.2019.00336. PMID: 31105512; PMCID: PMC6491889.*

80. *Culver A, Coiffard B, Antonini F, Duclos G, Hammad E, Vigne C, Mege JL, Baumstarck K, Boucekine M, Zieleskiewicz L, Leone M. Circadian disruption of core body temperature in trauma patients: a single-center retrospective observational study. J Intensive Care. 2020 Jan 6;8:4. doi: 10.1186/s40560-019-0425-x. PMID: 31921428; PMCID: PMC6945723.*

81. *Leung GKW, Huggins CE, Bonham MP. Effect of meal timing on postprandial glucose responses to a low glycemic index meal: A crossover trial in healthy volunteers. Clin Nutr. 2019 Feb;38(1):465-471. doi: 10.1016/j.clnu.2017.11.010. Epub 2017 Nov 22. PMID: 29248250.*

82. *Lévi F, Filipski E, Iurisci I, Li XM, Innominato P. Cross-talks between circadian timing system and cell division cycle determine cancer biology and therapeutics. Cold Spring Harb Symp Quant Biol. 2007;72:465-75. doi: 10.1101/sqb.2007.72.030. PMID: 18419306.*

83. *Chan K, Wong FS, Pearson JA. Circadian rhythms and pancreas physiology: A review. Front Endocrinol (Lausanne). 2022 Aug 10;13:920261. doi: 10.3389/fendo.2022.920261. PMID: 36034454; PMCID: PMC9399605.*

84. *Chan K, Wong FS, Pearson JA. Circadian rhythms and pancreas physiology: A review. Front Endocrinol (Lausanne). 2022 Aug 10;13:920261. doi: 10.3389/fendo.2022.920261. PMID: 36034454; PMCID: PMC9399605.*

85. *Elisabeth Filipski, Franck Delaunay, Verdun M. King, Ming-Wei Wu, Bruno Claustrat, Aline Grechez-Cassiau, Catherine Guettier, Michael H. Hastings, Levi Francis; Effects of Chronic Jet Lag on Tumor Progression in Mice. Cancer Res 1 November 2004; 64 (21): 7879–7885*

86. *Das M, Webster NJG. Obesity, cancer risk, and time-restricted eating. Cancer Metastasis Rev. 2022 Sep;41(3):697-717. doi: 10.1007/s10555-022-10061-3. Epub 2022 Aug 19. PMID: 35984550; PMCID: PMC9470651.*

87. *Chevalier G, Sinatra ST, Oschman JL, Sokal K, Sokal P. Earthing: health implications of reconnecting the human body to the Earth's surface electrons. J Environ Public Health. 2012;2012:291541. doi: 10.1155/2012/291541. Epub 2012 Jan 12. PMID: 22291721; PMCID: PMC3265077.*

88. *Chia-Jui Weng, Gow-Chin Yen, Chemopreventive effects of dietary phytochemicals against cancer invasion and metastasis: Phenolic acids, monophenol, polyphenol, and their derivatives, Cancer Treatment Reviews, Volume 38, Issue 1, 2012, Pages 76-87, ISSN 0305-7372,*

89. *Coiffard B, Diallo AB, Mezouar S, Leone M, Mege JL. A Tangled Threesome: Circadian Rhythm, Body Temperature Variations, and the Immune System. Biology (Basel). 2021 Jan 18;10(1):65. doi: 10.3390/biology10010065. PMID: 33477463; PMCID: PMC7829919.*

90. *Wright KP Jr, Hull JT, Czeisler CA. Relationship between alertness, performance, and body temperature in humans. Am J Physiol Regul Integr Comp Physiol. 2002 Dec;283(6):R1370-7. doi: 10.1152/ajpregu.00205.2002. Epub 2002 Aug 15. PMID: 12388468.*

CHAPTER -2

Haemoglobin & Cancer Connection

(Followed from rule-1 of chapter-1)

Let us now understand the connection and correlation between anemia and cancer. Here it goes!

Anemia causes tumor hypoxia, which often leads to Angiogenesis. As a result of Angiogenesis, the tumor aggressiveness increases. This condition is regarded as cancer.

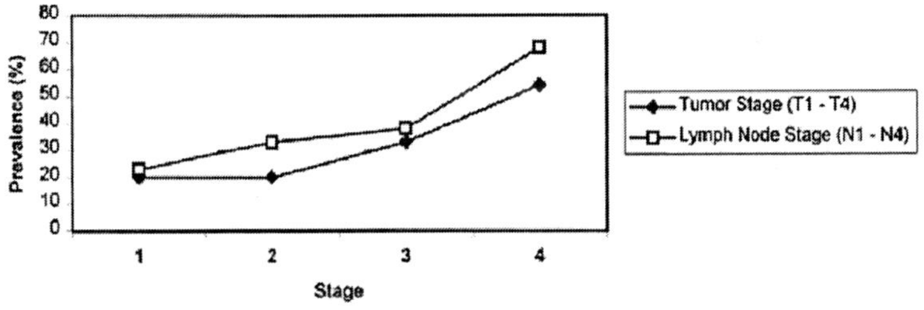

Prevalence of anemia by tumor and lymph node stages in patients with head and neck cancers. Anemia prevalence increases with disease severity, rising 3-fold from the earliest to the most advanced tumor stage and slightly less to the most advanced lymph node stage.[1]

As you can see in the table given below, whether it is the lung cancer, breast cancer, ovarian cancer or the cancer of the uterine cervix, leukemia, bone cancer, and even the Non-Hodgkin's Lymphoma and pancreatic cancer. On an average 90% of the patients, towards the end-stage of the cancer also suffer from anemia.

84% of patients with lung cancer had anemia.
82% of patients with breast cancer had anemia.
85% of patients with ovarian cancer had anemia.
93% of pancreatic cancer had anemia[2]

93% of patients with lymphoma had anemia.
97% of pediatric patients with leukemia had anemia.
78% of the bone cancer patient were found anemic.[3]

The correlation between anemia and cancer can also be concluded from the graph given below which shows the evidence of anemia by disease prevalence in patients with renal cancer.

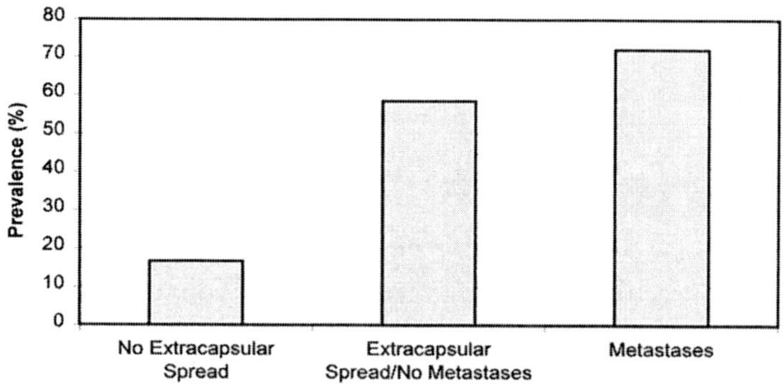

Prevalence of anemia by disease-severity in patients with renal cancer! Anemia prevalence increases about 4-fold with extracapsular spread and grows further with metastasis.[4]

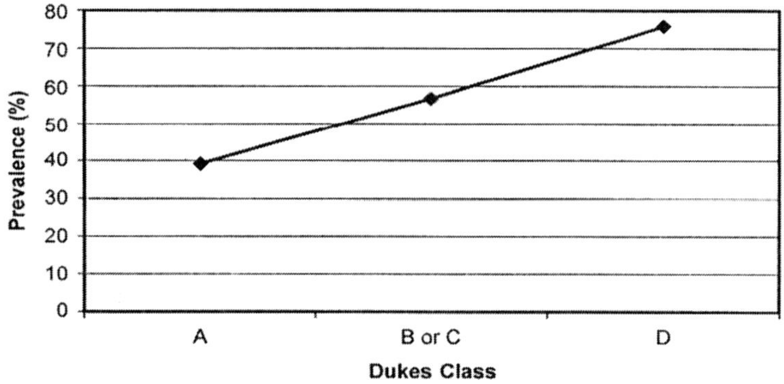

Prevalence of anemia in hospitalized patients with colon cancer varies with disease severity: 40% of patients with Dukes stage A tumors had anemia, compared with nearly 80% of patients with stage D tumors.[5]

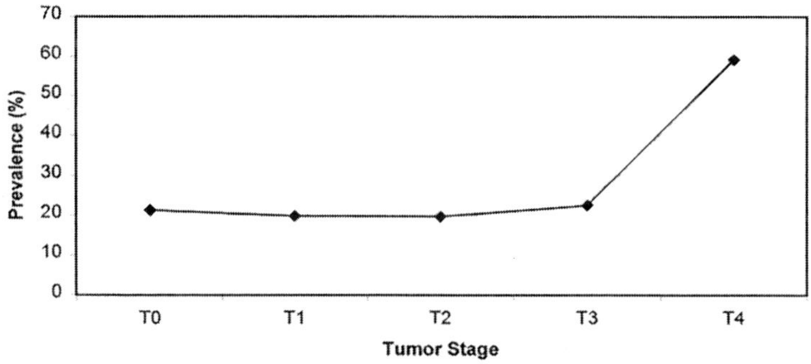

Prevalence of anemia in patients with prostate cancer appears relatively stable at about 20% in stages T0–T3; progression to stage T4 is associated with a 3-fold increase in prevalence.[6]

We can interpret this direct relation between anemia and end-stage cancer as a ray of hope. This means logically if we could remove anemia or increase the haemoglobin level in the body of the cancer patient, chances of the survival and of improving the quality of life of the patient should also proportionately improve as is suggested from various clinical studies.

The cross-sectional study reported an association between anemia and both functional and well-being scores.[7]

This suggests that if you wish to cure a cancer patient, then you must focus on the most important aspect of removing all those factors that result in an anemic condition, reduce the hemoglobin levels, or result in the destruction of RBC in the body. One of the major factors is the destruction of the circadian clock of red blood cells.[61] In the subsequent chapters you will learn about correcting the circadian clock.

As you would know that the treatment prescribed for cancer in modern medicine is chemotherapy and radiation. However, in reality both chemotherapy and radiation lead to anemia and destruction of RBCs in the body. In addition, both lead to the reduction of haemoglobin levels in the body. One can argue that chemotherapy as well as radiation procedures result in a dangerously uncontrolled reduction in haemoglobin in the system.

Prevalence of anemia in patients with cervical cancer was 67% before radiation therapy and 82% afterwards.[8]

In any respect, neither chemotherapy nor radiation is given to a patient to cure, control, or even prevent the cancer growth in the body. It is rather a mode to help the cancer spread throughout the system. I have been communicating about the adverse effects of chemotherapy and radiation to all my patients over the last several years. As you can see the references are provided in the boxes. All the references given below conclude only one thing that chemotherapy is not a cure for cancer, but promotes cancer growth in the patient's body.

Blood Health:
Chemotherapy decreases red blood cells (anemia)[9]
Chemotherapy decreases white blood cells (leukopenia)[10]
Chemotherapy decreases blood platelets [11]

Bone Health:
Chemotherapy causes bone death (osteonecrosis) [12]
Chemotherapy causes loss of bone mineral density (osteoporosis)[13-14]

Brain Health:
Chemotherapy is toxic to the brain (neurotoxic) [15]
Chemotherapy causes long-lasting impairment of concentration, forgetfulness and slower thinking; termed "chemobrain [16-17]
Chemotherapy causes altered consciousness [18]
Chemotherapy causes degeneration of white matter in the brain(leukoencephalopathy)[18]
Chemotherapy causes damage(neuropathy)[18]
Chemotherapy causes seizures [18]
Chemotherapy causes paralysis[18]
Chemotherapy causes stroke (cerebral infarction)[18]

Digestive Health:
Chemotherapy causes diarrhoea[26]
Chemotherapy causes painful inflammation and ulceration in the digestive tract (intestinal mucositis) [31]
Chemotherapy causes "significant intestinal damage in both jejunum and colon" [27]

Exercise:
Chemotherapy reduces grip strength[28]
Chemotherapy causes muscle dysfunction and a loss of overall strength[29]

Eye Health:
Chemotherapy causes severe vision loss and altered colorvision[30
Chemotherapy causes complete blindness[31]

Hair Health:
Chemotherapy causes hair-loss [38]

Healing:
Chemotherapy impairs wound healing [39]

Hearing:
Chemotherapy causes "severe to profound hearing loss"[40]
Chemotherapy causes chronic ringing of the ears (tinnitus)[40]

Heart Health:
Chemotherapy damages the heart[41]
Chemotherapy causes heart disease[42]
Chemotherapy causes heart failure[43]
Chemotherapy causes heart attacks (myocardial infarction)[44]

Immune System:
Chemotherapy causes long-term immune system damage [45-46]
Chemotherapy exacerbates existing hepatitis C infections[47]
Chemotherapy reactivates hepatitis B virus [48]
Chemotherapy impairs anti-tumor immune response [49]

Kidney Health:
Chemotherapy causes kidney failure [50]

Liver Health:
Chemotherapy causes liver injury [51]
Lung Health:
Chemotherapy causes lung disease[52]

Mental Health:
Chemotherapy "decreased emotional and social function and increased distress"[19]
Chemotherapy causes depression [20]

Chemotherapy causes anxiety [21]

Oral Health:

Chemotherapy causes severe dental caries [22]
Chemotherapy causes dry mouth (xerostomia), ulcers and mouth sores[53]
Chemotherapy causes oral candida (fungal) infection [23]
Chemotherapy causes painful inflammation and ulceration in the mouth (oral mucositis)[24]
Chemotherapy causes "a diverse spectrum of oral changes that generally are attributed to immunosuppression and bleeding tendencies" [25]

Pain:

Chemotherapy causes neuropathic pain; burning or coldness, "pins and needles" sensations, numbness and itching [54]
Chemotherapy pain remains one-year after treatment [55]

Quality of Life:

Chemotherapy causes diffculty swallowing (dysphagia) [56]
Chemotherapy causes nausea and vomiting (emesis) [57-58]
Chemotherapy causes altered taste sensation [59]
Chemotherapy causes migraine headaches [60]

Sexual Health:

Chemotherapy causes infertility and premature ovarian failure [32-33] in up to 66% of women [34]
Chemotherapy causes absence of menstrual period (amenorrhea) [35]
Chemotherapy causes menopausal symptoms[35]
Chemotherapy damages sperm and testicular tissue[36-37]
Chemotherapy reduces reproductive organ weight; sperm count and sperm motility[36]

References:

1. *Dubray B, Mosseri V, Brunin F, et al. Anemia is associated with lower local-regional control and survival after radiationtherapy for head and neck cancer: a prospective study. Radiology. 1996;201:553–558.*

2. *Tchekmedyian NS. Anemia in cancer patients: significance, epidemiology, and current therapy. Oncology (Huntingt). 2002;16(suppl 10):17–24.*

3. *Michon J. Incidence of anemia in pediatric cancer patients in Europe: results of a large, international survey. Med PediatrOncol. 2002;39:448–450.*

4. *vonKnorring J, Selroos O, Scheinin TM. Haematologic findings in patients with renal carcinoma.Scand J UrolNephrol. 1981;15:279–283.*

5. *Cappell MS, Goldberg ES. The relationship between the clinical presentation and spread of colon cancer in 315 consecutive patients: a significant trend of earlier cancer detection from 1982 through 1988 at a university hospital. J ClinGastroenterol. 1992;14:227–235.*

6. *Dunphy EP, Petersen IA, Cox RS, Bagshaw MA. The influence of initial hemoglobin and blood pressure levels on results of radiation therapy for carcinoma of the prostate. Int J RadiatOncolBiol Phys. 1989;16:1173–1178.*

7. *Cella D. The Functional Assessment of Cancer TherapyAnemia (FACT-An) Scale: a new tool for the assessment of outcomes in cancer anemia and fatigue. SeminHematol. 1997;34(suppl 2):13–19.*

8. *Harrison LB, Shasha D, White C, Ramdeen B. Radiotherapy-associated anemia: the scope of the problem. Oncologist. 2000;5(suppl 2):1–7.*

9. *Mountzios G, Aravantinos G, Alexopoulou Z, et al. Lessons from the past: Long-term safety and survival outcomes of a prematurely terminated randomized controlled trial on prophylactic vs. hemoglobin-based administration of erythropoiesis-stimulating agents in patients with chemotherapy-induced anemia. Mol Clin Oncol. 2016;4(2):211-220.*

10. *Li DY, Yu TT, Bai H, Chen XY. [Clinical study on effect of compound granule prescription of thunberg fritillary bulb in relieving post-chemotherapy bone marrow suppression in RAL patients]. Zhongguo Zhong Yao Za Zhi. 2012;37(20):3155-7.*

11. *Tamamyan G, Danielyan S, Lambert MP. Chemotherapy induced thrombocytopenia in pediatric oncology. Crit Rev Oncol Hematol. 2016;99:299-307.*

12. *Antonuzzo L, Lunghi A, Giommoni E, Brugia M, Di costanzo F. Regorafenib Also Can Cause Osteonecrosis of the Jaw. J Natl Cancer Inst. 2016;108(4).*

13. *Bordbar MR, Haghpanah S, Dabbaghmanesh MH, Omrani GR, Saki F. Bone mineral density in children with acute leukemia and its associated factors in Iran: a case-control study. Arch Osteoporos. 2016;11(1):36.*

14. *Lee SW, Yeo SG, Oh IH, Yeo JH, Park DC. Bone mineral density in women treated for various types of gynecological cancer. Asia Pac J Clin Oncol. 2016;*

15. *Matsuoka A, Mitsuma A, Maeda O, et al. Quantitative assessment of chemotherapy-induced peripheral neurotoxicity using a point-of-care nerve conduction device. Cancer Sci. 2016;107(10):1453-1457.*

16. *Iarkov A, Appunn D, Echeverria V. Post-treatment with cotinine improved memory and decreased depressive-like behavior after chemotherapy in rats. Cancer Chemother Pharmacol. 2016;78(5):1033-1039.*

17. *Rendeiro C, Sheriff A, Bhattacharya TK, et al. Long-lasting impairments in adult neurogenesis, spatial learning and memory from a standard chemotherapy regimen used to treat breast cancer. Behav Brain Res. 2016;315:10-22.*

18. *Reddy AT, Witek K. Neurologic complications of chemotherapy for children with cancer. Curr Neurol Neurosci Rep. 2003;3(2):137-42.*

19. *Dunn J, Watson M, Aitken JF, Hyde MK. Systematic Review of Psychosocial Outcomes for Patients with Advanced Melanoma. Psychooncology. 2016.*

20. *Oh PJ, Lee JR. [Effect of Cancer Symptoms and Fatigue on Chemotherapy-related Cognitive Impairment and Depression in People with Gastrointestinal Cancer). J Korean Acad Nurs. 2016;46(3):420-30.*

21. *Baek Y, Yi M. [Factors Influencing Quality of Life during Chemotherapy for Colorectal Cancer Patients in South Korea). J Korean Acad Nurs. 2015;45(4):604-12.*

22. *Peretz B, Sarnat H, Kharouba J. Chemotherapy induced dental changes in a child with medulloblastoma: a case report. J Clin Pediatr Dent. 2014;38(3):251-4.*

23. *Alt-epping B, Nejad RK, Jung K, Gross U, Nauck F. Symptoms of the oral cavity and their association with local microbiological and clinical findings–a prospective survey in palliative care. Support Care Cancer. 2012;20(3):531-7.*

24. *Dreizen S, Mccredie KB, Keating MJ. Chemotherapyinduced oral mucositis in adult leukemia. Postgrad Med. 1981;69(2):103-8, 111-2.*

25. *Farsi DJ. Children Undergoing Chemotherapy: Is It Too Late for Dental Rehabilitation?. J Clin Pediatr Dent. 2016;40(6):503-505.*

26. *Abalo R, Uranga JA, Pérez-garcía I, et al. May cannabinoids prevent the development of chemotherapy-induced diarrhea and intestinal mucositis? Experimental study in the rat. Neurogastroenterol Motil. 2016.*

27. *Forsgård RA, Korpela R, Holma R, et al. Intestinal permeability to iohexol as an in vivo marker of chemotherapy-induced gastrointestinal toxicity in SpragueDawley rats. Cancer Chemother Pharmacol. 2016;78(4):86374.*

28. *Klepin HD, Tooze JA, Pardee TS, et al. Effect of Intensive Chemotherapy on Physical, Cognitive, and Emotional Health of Older Adults with Acute Myeloid Leukemia. J Am Geriatr Soc. 2016;64(10):1988-1995.*

29. *Gilliam LA, Lark DS, Reese LR, et al. Targeted overexpression of mitochondrial catalase protects against cancer chemotherapy-induced skeletal muscle dysfunction. Am J Physiol Endocrinol Metab. 2016;311(2):E293-301.*

30. *Giralt J, Rey A, Villanueva R, Alforja S, Casaroli-marano RP. Severe visual loss in a breast cancer patient on chemotherapy. Med Oncol. 2012;29(4):2567-9.*

31. *Cloutier AO. Ocular side effects of chemotherapy: nursing management. Oncol Nurs Forum. 1992;19(8):1251-9.*

32 *Batchvarov IS, Taylor RW, Bustamante-marín X, et al. A grafted ovarian fragment rescues host fertility after chemotherapy. Mol Hum Reprod. 2016.*

33. *Clowse ME, Behera MA, Anders CK, et al. Ovarian preservation by GnRH agonists during chemotherapy: a meta-analysis. J Womens Health (Larchmt). 2009;18(3):3119.*

34. *Garrido-oyarzun MF, Castelo-branco C. Controversies over the use of GnRH agonists for reduction of chemotherapyinduced gonadotoxicity. Climacteric. 2016;19(6):522-525.*

35. *Li CY, Chen ML. [Chemotherapy-Induced Amenorrhea and Menopause Symptoms in Women With Breast Cancer). Hu Li Za Zhi. 2016;63(5):19-26.*

36. *Eid AH, Abdelkader NF, Abd el-raouf OM, Fawzy HM, Eldenshary ES. Carvedilol alleviates testicular and spermatological damage induced by cisplatin in rats via modulation of oxidative stress and inflammation. Arch Pharm Res. 2016.*

37. *Levi M, Popovtzer A, Tzabari M, et al. Cetuximab intensifies cisplatin-induced testicular toxicity. Reprod Biomed Online. 2016;33(1):102-10.*

38. Trüeb RM. Chemotherapy-induced alopecia. Semin Cutan Med Surg. 2009;28(1):11-4.

39. Tanaka S, Hayek G, Jayapratap P, et al. The Impact of Chemotherapy on Complications Associated with Mastectomy and Immediate Autologous Tissue Reconstruction. Am Surg. 2016;82(8):713-7.

40. Frisina RD, Wheeler HE, Fossa SD, et al. Comprehensive Audiometric Analysis of Hearing Impairment and Tinnitus After Cisplatin-Based Chemotherapy in Survivors of AdultOnset Cancer. J Clin Oncol. 2016;34(23):2712-20.

41. Truong J, Yan AT, Cramarossa G, Chan KK. Chemotherapy induced cardiotoxicity: detection, prevention, and management. Can J Cardiol. 2014;30(8):869-78.

42. Granger CB. Prediction and prevention of chemotherapy induced cardiomyopathy: can it be done?. Circulation. 2006;114(23):2432-3.

43. Smith SA, Auseon AJ. Chemotherapy-induced takotsubo cardiomyopathy. Heart Fail Clin. 2013;9(2):233-42.

44. Sakka S, Kawai K, Tsujimoto I, et al. [Severe Acute Myocardial Infarction during Induction Chemotherapy for Retroperitoneal Germ Cell Tumor : A Case Report]. Hinyokika Kiyo. 2016;62(9):483-487.

45. Perkins JL, Harris A, Pozos TC. Immune Dysfunction After Completion of Childhood Leukemia Therapy. J Pediatr Hematol Oncol. 2016.

46. Verma R, Foster RE, Horgan K, et al. Lymphocyte depletion and repopulation after chemotherapy for primary breast cancer. Breast Cancer Res. 2016;18(1):10.

47. Lin JW, Chang ML, Hsu CW, et al. Acute exacerbation of hepatitis C in hepatocellular carcinoma patients receiving chemotherapy. J Med Virol. 2017;89(1):153-160.

48. Qin L, Wang F, Zou BW, Ding ZY. Chemotherapy-induced fatal hepatitis B virus reactivation in a small-cell lung cancer patient. Mol Clin Oncol. 2016;5(4):382-384.

49. Wu Y, Deng Z, Wang H, Ma W, Zhou C, Zhang S. Repeated cycles of 5-fluorouracil chemotherapy impaired anti-tumour functions of cytotoxic T cells in a CT26 tumour-bearing mouse model. BMC Immunol. 2016;17(1):29.

50. Dugbartey GJ, Peppone LJ, De graaf IA. An integrative view of cisplatin-induced renal and cardiac toxicities: Molecular mechanisms, current treatment challenges and potential protective measures. Toxicology. 2016;371:58-66.

51. *Hiroshima Y, Shuto K, Yamazaki K, et al. Fractal Dimension of Tc-99m DTPA GSA Estimates Pathologic Liver Injury due to Chemotherapy in Liver Cancer Patients. Ann Surg Oncol. 2016;23(13):4384-4391.*

52. *Limper AH. Chemotherapy-induced lung disease. Clin Chest Med. 2004;25(1):53-64.*

53. *Berger velten D, Zandonade E, Monteiro de barros miotto MH. Prevalence of oral manifestations in children and adolescents with cancer submitted to chemotherapy. BMC Oral Health. 2016;16(1):107.*

54. *Gong SS, Li YX, Zhang MT, et al. Neuroprotective Effect of Matrine in Mouse Model of Vincristine-Induced Neuropathic Pain. Neurochem Res. 2016;41(11):3147-3159.*

55. *Hellerstedt-börjesson S, Nordin K, Fjällskog ML, Holmström IK, Arving C. Women Treated for Breast Cancer Experiences of Chemotherapy-Induced Pain: Memories, Any Present Pain, and Future Reflections. Cancer Nurs. 2016;39(6):464472.*

56. *Mcnamara MJ, Adelstein DJ, Allende DS, et al. Persistent Dysphagia After Induction Chemotherapy in Patients with Esophageal Adenocarcinoma Predicts Poor Post-Operative Outcomes. J Gastrointest Cancer. 2016.*

57. *Fakhfouri G, Mousavizadeh K, Mehr SE, et al. From Chemotherapy-Induced Emesis to Neuroprotection: Therapeutic Opportunities for 5-HT3 Receptor Antagonists. Mol Neurobiol. 2015;52(3):1670-9.*

58. *Thamlikitkul L, Srimuninnimit V, Akewanlop C, et al. Efficacy of ginger for prophylaxis of chemotherapy-induced nausea and vomiting in breast cancer patients receiving adriamycin-cyclophosphamide regimen: a randomized, double-blind, placebo-controlled, crossover study. Support Care Cancer. 2016.*

59. *Sozeri E, Kutluturkan S. The Validity and Reliability of Turkish Version of the Chemotherapy-induced Taste Alteration Scale (CITAS). Clin Nurs Res. 2016.*

60. *Rajasekhar A, George TJ. Gemcitabine-induced reversible posterior leukoencephalopathy syndrome: a case report and review of the literature. Oncologist. 2007;12(11):1332-5.*

61. *O'Neill JS, Reddy AB. Circadian clocks in human red blood cells. Nature. 2011 Jan 27;469(7331):498-503. doi: 10.1038/nature09702. PMID: 21270888; PMCID: PMC3040566.*

CHAPTER -3

How To Invent a Cancer Patient?

(Followed from rule-2 of chapter-1)

Let us understand, when a doctor refers to a patient as stage I, II, III or IV cancer, what do they mean? Stage I: The cancer is localized to a small area and hasn't spread to lymph nodes or other tissues. Stage II: The cancer has grown, but it hasn't spread. Stage III: The cancer has grown larger and has possibly spread to lymph nodes or other tissues. Stage IV: The cancer has spread to other organs or areas of the body. It should be noted that the decrease of stages is equivalent to the decrease in the spread of malignant cells over the affected area. There is a Stage Zero also for those people like you and me.

How does the doctor discover that the cancer has spread to how many parts of a body? There is a popular test that is considered very reliable in the medical circles – which is called the Positron Emission Tomography or PET Scan.

Now, let us discover what a PET scan is and how does this become the basis of detecting cancer. This is something you need to importantly understand for knowing the entire game around cancer industry.

Positron emission tomography or PET scan

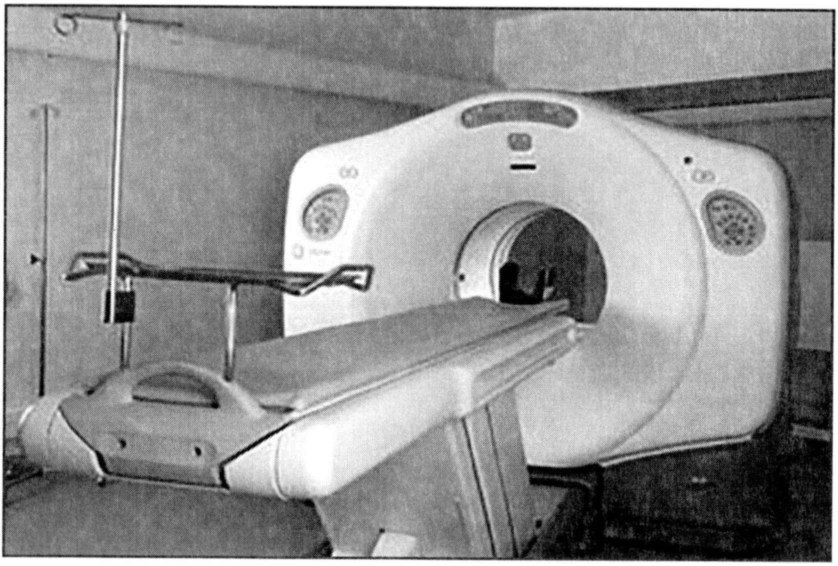

This picture shows the PET scan machinery in which the patient is asked to lie down (after injecting radioactive glucose/fluorodeoxyglucose in the body). This machine will take certain pictures of various parts of your body to find out the growth of cancer cells. These images and films will now reveal certain bright and shining spots that the machine had scanned. As per the theory or assumption, the over-active brighter cells are cancer cells therefore, your body cells that are over-active and brighter than the rest of the cells will be termed as cancer. Remember that anyone's cells that become more active consume more energy or sugar than the rest of the cells.

Let us take the current instance of your reading my book right now. Now your body cells that are engaged in reading are more active and alive, which means these cells are consuming extra energy. All cells utilize energy from glucose in human body but those that are consuming more glucose only mean they are engaged in extra work and therefore, working harder than the rest of the cells. However, the cells after doing PET scans are termed to be cancerous, even though they might just be over-worked due to some extra hard-work. It is just like saying that those children who consume more food in a day than the rest are comparatively naughtier or else, those children who eat less are less naughty. Yes, there may be a possibility that some kids eat more and are indeed naughtier than the rest of the kids but opposite can also be true. There may be some children who eat less and are naughtier than those who eat more.

There could be many instances to prove that there are many cells in our body that consume less sugar but grow at a fast rate or are over-active. Therefore, the over-active cells are cancerous - is just a basic assumption that does not have a scientific basis. On the other hand, it is also scientifically disapproved but unfortunately this is the basis of PET scan diagnosis. Just like the theory related to more food and naughtier children cannot be ascertained, likewise, the theory of more over-active cells and images of shiny clusters found in PET scans rule out the probability of cancer. [1,2]

So how does the doctor go about such procedures of scanning the cancer cells? Or else, how does he know how many cells are consuming more sugar in the body. So, there is a scanning procedure in order to find this out. At first, the patients are asked to go on a complete fasting or at least for an 18-hour fasting. Fasting would result in all the cells of the body going hungry and cells are now waiting for glucose. Once over with the fasting, instead of giving normal glucose to the body, the doctors will inject the body with something called or Fluorodeoxyglucose, commonly known as FDGs.

Fluorodeoxyglucose (FDG)

FDGs are a radioactive material with one part glucose. Since the body is already on fast and also hungry, the FDGs will be quickly absorbed by the body cells. Those cells that are hungrier than the rest will naturally absorb more FDGs. As a result, those cells, being already inserted with radio-active materials will therefore shine out and be brighter in the images taken by PET scan machine. On the basis of such images that are found over-active and shining cells, the doctors will ascertain that you are a cancer patient.

In the two sets of images given below you will clearly notice the shining spots. The abdomen in the first image and the shoulder plus abdomen in the second image clearly shows the shining cells. The doctor will now indicate that the cancer cells are spread to quite an extent as shown via these bright spots. This could be fourth stage of cancer as per the doctor. The reality, however, they may just be those cells that consume more sugar are shining more brightly than the rest. There may be multiple reasons why certain cells would consume more sugar than the rest.[3]

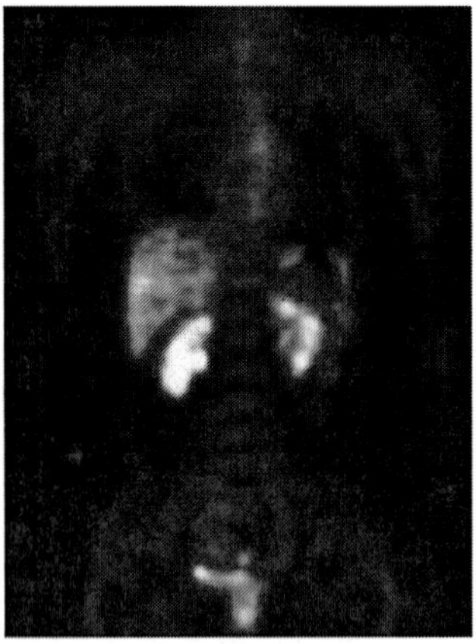

PET Scan (Abdomen)

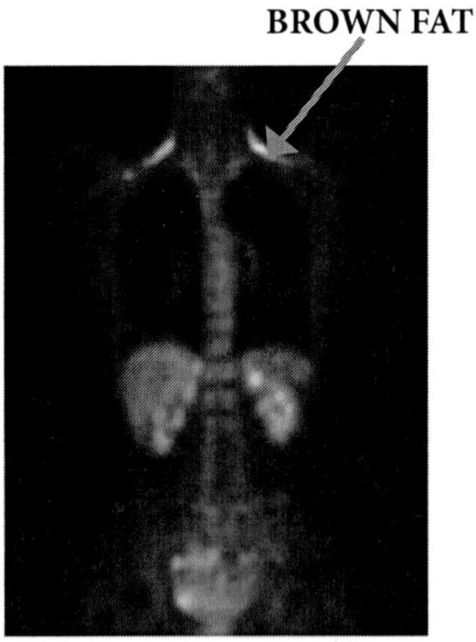

PET Scan (Shoulder)

In this image, we can notice some areas on the shoulder which is called the 'brown fat'. The basic function of brown fat is to control the thermodynamics of the body or in simple terms, control the heat system of the body. During winter times, we shiver and in turn, we generate heat in the body. All this is with the help of brown fat that is found on the shoulders and neck region. So, in case you are less on body fat, or thin, or facing wintry conditions, this brown fat will help you with body heat generation. In such a scenario, the PET scan will show you more bright spots. This certainly does not mean you have cancer. [4]

Another important example is our Thyroid gland that is a source of consuming lots of sugar/glucose due to its nature of functionality. Just as a Mercedes Car operates on more fuel consumption compared with a car like Maruti 800 due to its engine size and functionality, thyroid glands too consume more glucose and energy. This is why up to one-third persons who are PET scanned are detected with mimicking cancer, whereas this is just a depiction of thyroid sugar consumption. So, the brown fat cells that have more active mitochondria consume more sugar or thyroid glands that have more brightness in PET scans cannot be termed as cancer.[4] This kind of hypothesis on cancer is unscientific.

Serum Uptake Value (SUV)

Similarly, there is another criteria used to determine cancer cells. This is based on a calculation of how much Fluorodeoxyglucose or FDGs were absorbed by your cells. In this calculation there is a random number of 2.5 Serum Uptake Value or SUVs that is consumed by the cells becomes a criteria for notifying cancerous cells. Brown fat cells sometimes show 3 or 4 SUV count and thyroid glands show 7 or 10 SUV count despite functioning normally.[5] In such a case, when the patient approaches another doctor for a second opinion with such reports, he or she again receives similar opinion. Since all the doctors belong to the same community, most doctors will read the diagnosis in the same way and make sure the patient also starts feeling the same. So, the person who is not even a patient will now become a cancer patient.

Irritable Bowel Syndrome (IBS)

Another example is that of IBS or those who have irritable bowel syndrome. These patients have a tendency of having such microbes in their stomach that consume more sugar. When such patients suffering from IBS would go for PET scan they will be falsely detected with cancer too.[6] In other words, if such a patient goes for PET Scan, he will be told that he is suffering from abdomen cancer. Similarly, those suffering from the Auto Immune diseases or those patients who have certain plaques or blockages in their body are prone to be diagnosed by the doctors wrongly as cancer patients. [7]

Another area of bodily suffering is infection inside the body or sores then the inflammatory cells of the body that normally function towards fighting off the infection and repair the damaged cells wherever there is injury. Naturally such activities will have more energy consumption around it and therefore an increased FDG uptake will be found in such regions. The doctors will predict this to be cancer. [8] Moving to another interesting area is Vascular Endothelial Growth Factor or VEGF which is a special molecule that acts as a middle-man in the body with a function to bring a balance to the over-active as well as under-active cells of the body. Whenever this molecule will start its function, it will consume more glucose than the rest. [9]

PET scan false diagnosis due to:

1. Brown fat

2. Thyroid

3. IBS

4. Auto immune disease

5. Plaque
6. Infection
7. Inflammatory cells
8. VEGF
9. Healing tissue/bones

So, all kinds of repairing carried out inside the body is termed as cancer by PET scan. An important thing to notice is that PET scan never diagnoses that your body has cancer or not but this scan only diagnoses about which cells are consuming more sugar at a given point of time. So, it does not necessarily mean that the same cells will consume more sugar in future or not.[10] Once these cells in the healing tissues and bones are completely healed the sugar consumption will automatically decrease.[11]

Let me suggest an experiment at this point that can be done at home too – in order to understand the previously discussed points. When you are ready to go for a PET scan, you can manipulate your reports by following my suggestions.

Activities that enhance sugar uptake by cells:
1. Muscle Activity
2. Speech
3. Non fasting
4. Mensuration cycle/Ovulation day
5. Testosterone production
6.Lactating mother

1. Arm exercises

You can perform dumbbells or weights (used in gym) exercise for 15 minutes. And after an hour go for PET scan.[10] Once you do this exercise, your arm tissues and cells will be hungry for some extra sugar. Now when the PET scan is carried out, your doctor will likely suggest a tumor in your arm. It was just a case of exercising and additional amount of sugar requirement by the arm muscles.

Take another example of small children. All those who have small children would know that the hunger of children depends on several factors such as what mood the child is in or what is the favorite food of the child, else the child has eaten something already, or may be the child is suffering ill health, etc. Hence, there are many factors governing what and when will the child eat or how much will he or she eat. Food eating is variable depending on many factors. Similarly, our body cells also eat variably, depending on many factors.

2. Facial muscles and speech

While getting your PET scan done facial muscles and making a speech during the scan makes a big difference. If you are getting the PET scan done, also speak at the same time, your facial muscles will be activated. It is observed that in such cases, you may be told that you have oral cancer, as per the doctors. However, if you wish to reverse the result of PET scan, you just have to eat before this procedure. Now when the doctor will inject FDGs, the result will not show shining cells in the images as you have supplied the cells with enough glucose by eating. The doctor will now tell you that you no longer have cancer. [12]

Menstrual cycle

When the time of menstrual cycle and ovulation amongst women comes closer, the areas around uterus and ovaries become more active than normal. This is why the sugar uptake is more than normal during this time and therefore the FDG uptake may also be more than normal. At this time the doctors can wrongly diagnose that you have ovarian cancer or uterus cancer. Or else, in case you have ovarian cysts, the doctors can give you similar diagnosis. [13]

Testosterone

Similarly, as an experiment amongst males, just before the PET scan, if they are shown some erotic or pornographic material, the levels of testosterone will naturally increase in the blood as a result of which, the requirement of sugar increases in the testes.[14] In such a situation, when given a PET scan, the FDG uptake will also increase. The doctors can now claim that you have testicular cancer, whereas it was just a case of watching pornographic material.

Lactating mothers

At the time when mothers who are breast feeding their infants, their breast tissues and muscles become over active. At such times their requirement of sugar will be more than usual in this region. The doctor will now claim that you may have a chance of breast cancer. The logic is simply that metabolically, the breast is over active and the uptake of sugar and FDG is more than usual here. He will suggest biopsy or other related procedures. An important point to remember is that such procedures like biopsy can result in cancer growth. Biopsy is almost an invitation for cancer, is my suggestion to you all, so it is advisable to avoid such tests. I have already provided all kinds of evidences related to such topics in my book, "The case against IMA" that is available for you on the link - www.biswaroop.com/ebook. [15]

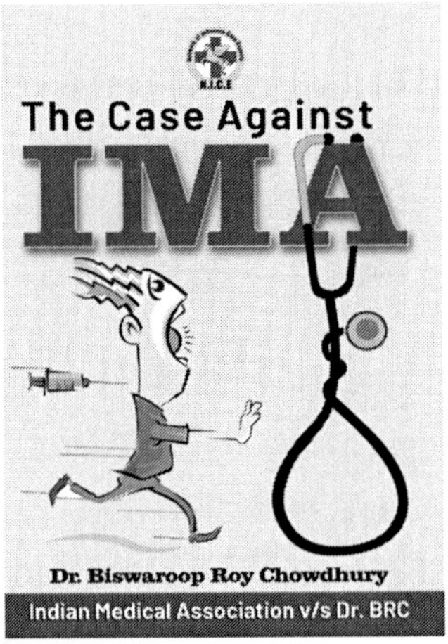

How doctors can manipulate your tests

We have discovered how you can manipulate the FDG results by carrying out experiments at your end, you should also note how doctors can manipulate your tests by certain means in order to certify that you are suffering from cancer.

1. **FDG Dose**
2. **Injected Clot**
3. **Insulin before PET scan**
4. **Radiation Induced**
5. **COVID – Vaccine**
6. **PSA**

Manipulating FDG dosage

The first amongst such manipulations is the quantity of FDG dose that needs to be given to the patient. Suppose the stipulated quantity is 350 and in order to see more shining spots, in the body, the doctor doubles the dose and makes it 700. It will naturally give more shine in the spots that denote cancerous areas. [16]

Injected clots

Another way of manipulation is the syringe usage. When the piston of this syringe that is inserted in your body, is pulled out of the body, when that blood is pushed back to the body as a clot, it will make a hot-spot. This kind of activity will increase the uptake of FDGs. According to the protocol set by cancer detection, this can be termed as cancer. [17]

Insulin intake before PET scan

Just before the PET scan, if the patient is provided an insulin intake, it is a fact that those cells that absorb the insulin tend to also absorb more FDGs than usual. So if as a doctor, I need to prove to you that you are suffering from cancer, I only need to tell the radiologist to inject some 15-20 units of insulin. Now your PET scan will give a report of your having cancer.

Radiation induced manipulation

At the beginning of this chapter, I had pointed out that FDG itself is a radioactive material. Most of us know that radiation is a serious cause of cancer. More so, it is clearly written in PET scan precaution that after getting a PET scan done for about a day you are not supposed to go near children or pregnant women.[18] This is because you are a walking talking radioactive material now and you can harm them clearly. It does not go without saying that when you are yourself carrying so much FDG inside your body, will you not end up having cancer?

Since it is clearly written in the PET scan precaution that after such a scan, your chances of having cancer will increase. Imagine how a healthy person injects himself or herself with poison and radiation, which is already known and written and then goes on to complain that he is a cancer patient. Now, do you think that the title: How to Invent a Cancer Patient, is justifiable?

COVID-vaccine

The most dangerous thing, the fifth one, is the covid vaccine.[19] Those who have taken two doses of covid vaccine and have gone for PET scan after that, the reports were altogether different. It has been proven by research papers[19] that in such cases they are more prone to be diagnosed as cancer patients.

PSA

There are many more widespread diagnostic methods to invent cancer patients. For instance, according to the discoverer of Prostate Specific

Antigen (PSA), Richard Ablin, the PSA test for cancer is no more accurate than the toss of a coin.[20] PSA level can be elevated by a number of factors such as ejaculation 24 hours prior to the test, an infection or activities that "massage the prostate", like a long bicycle ride.

So, cancer patients are not there but are made by these theories and the trap of diagnostic tests. I do not say that there are no cancer patients or there are no over-active cells but this is a trap. When patients come to me complaining of cancer, I ask them what are the problems they are facing, whether there is some pain, weakness, low-grade fever or any unusual symptoms, they say that they don't have any such problems but their PET scan shows that they have cancer. This means they have fallen in the trap. Now the question is – what to do?

First step is to diagnose whether your body has over-active cells. For this, remember five points:

Self-diagnosis of cancer

In order to conduct a safe diagnosis of cancer or to have a knowledge whether you have any over-active cells in your body, you need to enquire five points that may be a constant feature of your body:

1. It can be a constant weakness
2. Low grade fever that lasts for almost a month
3. Constant body-ache
4. Any unusual symptom in the body
5. Your hemoglobin consistently coming down.

If you have noticed any of these symptoms then you should understand that your body is having some overactive cell development. Now, how to get cured out of this serious situation. For that fix/reset your 'Circadian

Rhythm/body's clock, which may be out of control sometimes and leads to over-active cells. This will lead to all kinds of difficulties that is normally termed as cancer.[21]

Circadian Rhythm is explained in the next chapter.

References:

1. *Shreve PD, Anzai Y, Wahl RL: Pitfalls in Oncologic Diagnosis with FDG PET Imaging: Physiologic and Benign Variants, Radio Graphics: 1999;19 (1) : 61-77.*
2. *Lin E, Alavi A (2009) PET/CT: A Clinical Guide, 2nd Edition, Thieme Publications, New York, Pg. 145.*
3. *Alavi A, Gupta N, Alberini JL, Hickeson M, Adam LE, Bhargava P, et al : Positron Emission Tomography Imaging in non-malignant thoracic disorder; Semin Nucl Med 2002;32 : 293-321.*
4. *Truong MT, Erasmus JJ, Munden RF, Marom EM, Sabloffs BS, Gladish GW, Podoloff DA, Macapinlac HA : Focal FDG uptake in mediastinal brown fat mimicking malignancy: a potential pitfall resolved on PET/CT : Am J Roentgenol, 2004;183(4) : 1127- 1132.*
5. *Keyes JW Jr, SUV: standard uptake or silly useless value? J Nucl Med 1995;36:1836-1839.*
6. *Meyer MA. Diffused increased colonic F-18 FDG uptake in acutenterocolitis Clin Nuc Med 1995;20: 434-435.*
7. *Boerner AR, Voth E, Theissen P, Wienhard K, Wagner R, Schicha H: Glucose metabolism of the thyroid in Graves' disease measured by F-18 Fluoro-deoxyglucose positron emission tomography. Thyroid 1998-8-765-772.*
8. *Im JG, Kong Y, Shin YM, Yang SO, Song JG, Han MC, et al. Pulmonary paragonimiasis: clinical and experimental studies. Radiographics 1993:13:575-586.*

9. *Maschauer S, Prante O, Hoffman M, Deichen JT, Kuwert T. Characterisation of 18-FFDG uptake in human endothelial cells in vitro. J Nucl Med. 2004; 45:455-460.*

10. *Brigid GA, Flanagan FL, Dehdashti F. Whole body positron emission tomography: normal variations, pitfalls and technical considerations. AIR 1997; 169;1675-1680.*

11. *Meyer M, Gast T, Raja S. Hubnar K. Increased F-18 FDG accumulation in an Nishizawa S, Menstruation M, Okada H. Physiological 18F – FDG uptake in the ovaries and uterus of healthy female volunteers. Furl, Nucl Med Mol Imaging. December 2004.*

12. *Yeung HW, Grewal RK, Gonen M, Schöder H, Larson SM. Patterns of (18) F-FDG uptake in adipose tissue and muscle: a potential source of false-positives for PET. J NuclMed. 2003;44(11):1789–1796.*

13. *Nishizawa S, Menstruation M, Okada H. Physiological 18F – FDG uptake in the ovaries and uterus of healthy female volunteers. Furl, Nucl Med Mol Imaging. December 2004.*

14. *LH pulsatile secretion and testosterone blood levels are influenced by sexual arousal in human males. Psychoneuroendocrinology. 1993:18 (3). Doi: 10.1016/0306 -4530 (93)90005-6.*

15. *Kosuda S, Fischer S, Kison PV, Wahl RL, Grossman HB. Uptake 2-deoxy-2 –[18 F] fluoro-D-glucose in the normal testes : retrospective PET study and animal experiment.*

16. *Jones SC, Alavi A, Christman D, Montanez I, Wolf AP, Reivich M. The radiation dosimetry of 2-[F-18] fluoro-2-deoxy-Dglucose in man. J Nucl Med 1982; 23:613–617.*

17. *Lin E, Alavi A (2009) PET/CT: A Clinical Guide, 2nd Edition, Thieme Publications, New York, Pg. 145.*

18. *Lin P, Chu J, Pocock N. Fluorine -18 FDG dual-head gamma camera coincidence imaging of radiation pneumonitis. Clin Nucl Med 2000;25: 866-869.*

19. *COVID-19 Vaccination-Related Uptake on FDG PET/CT: An Emerging Dilemma and Suggestions for Management AJR Am J Roentgenol. 2021 Oct; 217(4) : 975-83.doi:10.2214/AJR.21.25728 .*

20. *Brett, Allan, MD, Prof., Dept. Clinical Internal Medicine, Univ. South Carolina School of Medicine, Columbia, SC. Against PSA screening; co-author with Richard J. Ablin, NEJM article United States Preventive Services Task Force recommendation (Brett and Ablin, NEJM, 365, 1949, 2011). May 10, 2013.*

21. *Interplay between Circadian Clock and Cancer: New Frontiers for Cancer Treatment Trends, 2019, Aug: 5(8); 475-494. Doi: 10.1016/j.trecan.2019.07.002.*

CHAPTER -4

Resetting Body Clock*

(Followed from rule-4 of chapter-1)

**Adapted from Lecture-2 of Zero Volt Therapy Certification Course*

How vital is the body clock for our good health can be understood with the fact that this theory of your circadian rhythm has received a Nobel Prize in Medicine, in 2017. The three American scientists who received the Nobel recognition for their discoveries in the mechanisms controlling the circadian rhythms are: Jeffery C Hall, Michael Rosbash and Michael Young, have detailed about the circadian rhythm and its effects on health.

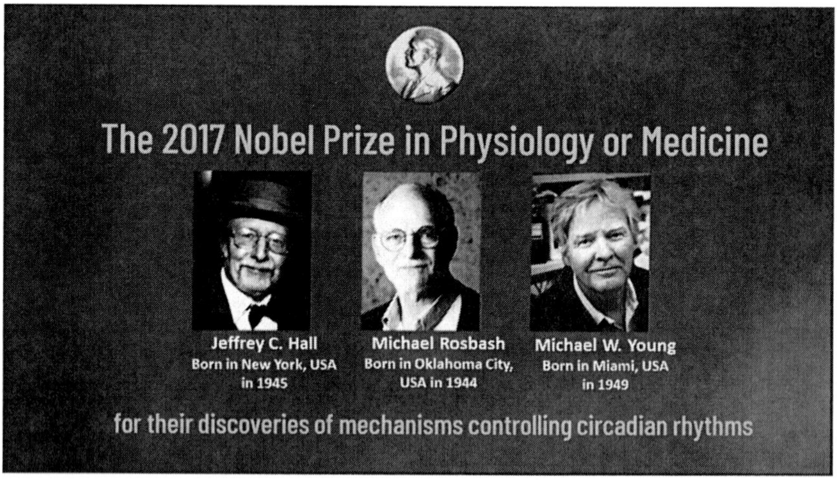
The 2017 Nobel Prize in Physiology or Medicine
Jeffrey C. Hall
Born in New York, USA in 1945
Michael Rosbash
Born in Oklahoma City, USA in 1944
Michael W. Young
Born in Miami, USA in 1949
for their discoveries of mechanisms controlling circadian rhythms

This means that when the body clock or your circadian rhythm gets disturbed, it produces all kinds of illness and the illness causes distraction or disturbance in your body clock.

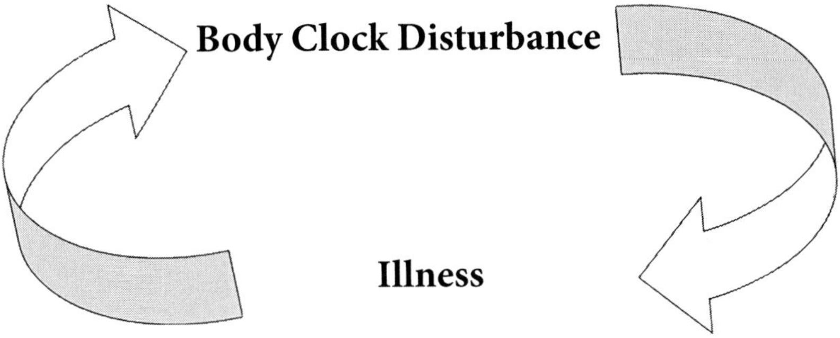

So this is a vicious cycle which means, whatever illness you may be suffering from – it can be cancer, heart disease, Parkinson or else tuberculosis, if you wish to cure your disease the best way is to correct your body clock or your circadian rhythm.

The Circadian Rhythm Cycle

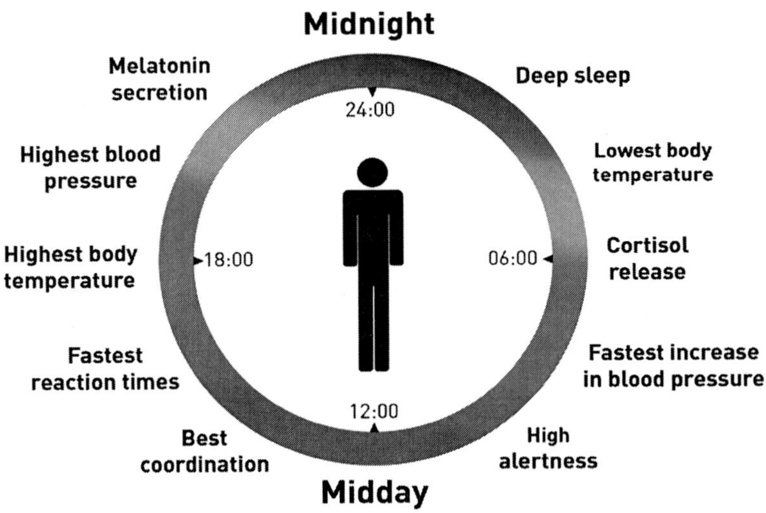

Understanding circadian rhytm

'Circadian rhythm' simply means your 'body clock'. Your body is designed for certain kinds of activities that are governed by certain secretions to be released at certain points of time in a period of 24 hours. For example, after sunset your body is designed to produce more melatonin, which helps you to sleep better. Similarly, when you get up in the morning, your body is expected to produce more cortisol, which helps you to remain active throughout the day. At night, your body is expected to produce lowest temperature. This way, body functions with certain kind of rules. In case, your body keeps up with these rules, your body will result in its highest performance. In case this rhythm is disturbed, let's say the melatonin is not produced at the right time or cortisol is not produced in the morning, there are chances that you will feel weak or dizzy and may be during the night you might feel more alert and not sleepy. This means that any disturbance in the circadian rhythm will attract illness or weakness.

Tools to fix the circadian rhythm

In order to correct your body clock, you need certain kind of tools. I shall give you three such tools that will help you achieve the right balance. These tools are very simple: light, time of eating and sleep.

Body Clock
1. Light **2. Time of eating** **3. Sleep**

Out of the three tools, the most interesting one is the light. This simple tool of light that is able to fix your circadian rhythm applies on any one and anywhere to help your body clock to function correctly.

First tool - Light

As per the research paper of K.P. Wright, Jr. et al, "Entrainment of the Human Circadian Clock to the Natural Light-Dark Cycle,"[1] we can understand that human body follows a light and dark cycle. During the 24-hour cycle, a part is sunrise and a part is sunset. This means that your body is balanced between living in darkness and light for a certain duration of time. However, after the times of electricity and bulb invention, we are exposed to light even after sun-set. This severely interferes with our body clock and disturbs the circadian rhythm.

A simple cure to this disturbance is that after sunrise, through the day you should be exposed at least half an hour to one hour of 1000 Lux of any kind of light. Similarly, after sunset, you need to be exposed to light 'not' more than 50 Lux. Once you maintain this, your body will experience a balanced clock.

After Sunrise	After Sunset
More than1000 Lux	Less than 50 Lux

Correcting Sleep

Measurement of light

In order to know how much is 50 Lux of light, we need to use the lux measuring instrument that comes with a light sensor attachment. As you will switch the instrument on, the digital display will automatically tell you the strength of light in the room. Further, if you bring the sensor closer to the light source, you will be able to check the measurement of light source too.

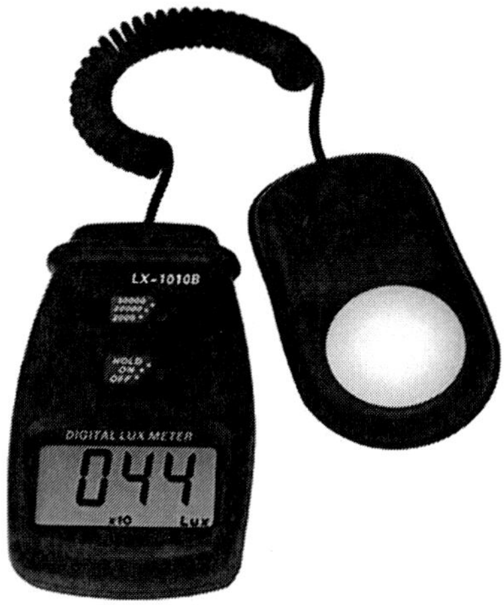

Lightmeter/Luxmeter

In all probability, some of you might be knowing that a bright source of light works better than having anti-depressant tablets. In case a patient gets to be exposed to 10,000 Lux of light for a period of 30 to 60 minutes, it will be equivalent to taking an anti-depressant tablet for those who feel low or depressed. This means the body needs at least this much amount of light to produce serotonin to be able to feel good.

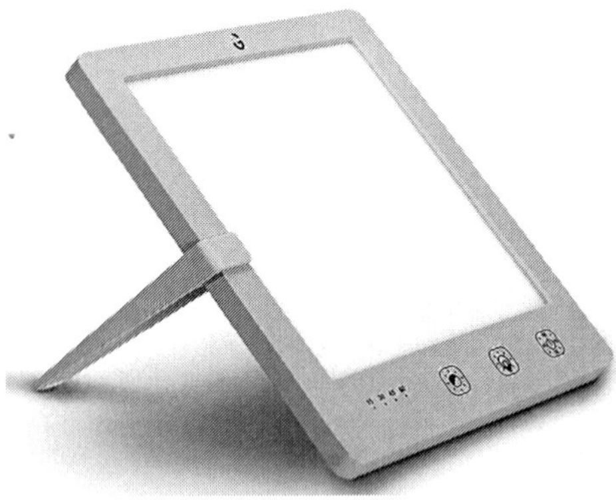

Light therapy lamp

However, if you get exposed to sunlight, the amount of light is equivalent to 1 to 3 lacs lux of light. You can check the same by downloading a lux measuring app that is downloadable on any android. Just Google for "Lux Meter – Light Meter" for downloading the app and you will not even need to buy the light meter. So now you must have understood the importance of light on human body that eventually controls your mood, sleep and overall health.

Google Play **Light Meter - Lux Meter**

Even in the past several years, researches have proven the connection between light and sleep. The studies proves that if you have two hours of dim light before sleeping, you will have a good sleep through the night. Similarly, the opposite is true during the day. If you are exposed to a good amount of daylight, your office performance during the day increases.

Daylight →Office performance Connection[2]

Also, scientists have discovered the disturbance in circadian clock due to LED lights at night. We are used to getting exposed to light emitting diodes (LED) that has resulted in various kinds of diseases due to its mal-effect on our body clock.

Dim nightlight →Sleep Connection[3]

Light as medicine

All such researches only go on to prove that light works as medicine or a drug. It helps the body to produce hormones congenial to the well-being of the body. However, if you are exposed to light at the wrong timing, it can work adversely, just like any other drug. This is especially true with children's brain being affected adversely by exposure to long hours to light after sunset. This is what has been noticed throughout the globe in the past three years after the COVID lockdown when everything was shifted online. As a result, they got more access to laptops and mobiles; also, due to watching television for a longer time, children were exposed to more light and even the harmful blue light during the night time.

The past two years have proven that the attention deficit / hyperactivity disorder (ADHD) amongst children have had an all-time rise throughout the world. This goes on to prove that there is a direct connection of children having ADHD with exposure to blue light.[4]

Evening LED light[5]

It also means that if you want to cure or even reverse a patient of ADHD, one way is that you need to balance the light in her/his system. You need to ensure that the child gets enough sunlight in the morning and through the day, whereas during the night, the child must not be exposed to the blue, bright or flashy light of TV or any other screen. This will give you very quick results in children and provide symptomatic relief to ADHD.

Medicine for ADHD[6]

Second tool - Timing of food

The second tool that fixes the circadian rhythm is 'timing of food intake'. In case you eat within a bracket of ten hours i.e., if you eat between 8:00 am in the morning and 6:00 pm in the evening and keep your food intake limited during this period, you will experience an immense relief in heart or liver diseases. I call this as a 10-hour diet rule that can cure many diseases within a few days.

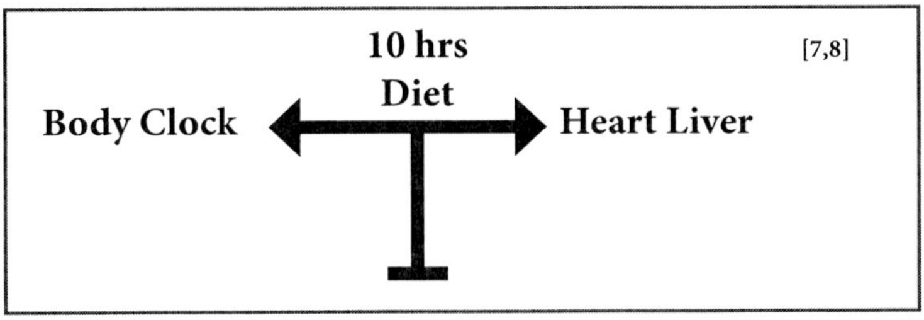

10 hour Diet rule[9, 10]

This simply means you are avoiding food for the rest of the 14-hour bracket. This 14-hour gap gives the body to change its setting by releasing more good bacteria in the gut. These good bacteria are responsible to produce hormones in the body that can cure many diseases. For instance, in the brain curing the nervous system or in the intestines and colon to control the insulin in your pancreatic system and similarly other things. This way the gut becomes the control room for the production of hormones in various parts of the body. Therefore, good bacteria production can be controlled by your eating habits and water fasting during the 14-hour period.

10 hour Diet rule[11]

8 Hrs * 8 weeks Diet Rule

The second tool that fixes your circadian rhythm also helps in losing weight. Now that is an interesting fact. Suppose you eat a particular amount of food, let's say 2 kgs of food, in a shorter window of 10 hours, it will help your body to gaining lesser weight. This is as against your intake of the same quantity of 2 kgs food over a longer span of duration - let's say 16 hours – that will allow your body to deposit more fat than it did over a 10-hour span.

Less window of eating = Less weight [12]

This way the same amount of food in the bigger bracket of time will save you from a number of diseases. On the other hand, if you consume the same food in lesser bracket of time, you can reverse diseases like heart disease, various metabolic diseases like hypertension, and diabetes and strength related issues.

8 hrs x 8 week Diet Rule[13,14]

- **Heart Disease**
- **Strength**
- **Metabolic Disorder**

You can take a 3-day challenge, where your diet remains the same as per quantity of food intake but you will only eat in the bracket of eight hours. Just by doing so, your blood sugar and blood pressure is expected to be in better control within 3 days. You can feel the difference yourself and if you continue the same for 8 weeks, your body clock is likely to correct itself, giving you a balanced circadian rhythm. This way, all the diseases in your body are expected to start vanishing. This will give you proof enough that your body clock re-fix will give you a better health. This means eating within a stipulated time frame works like a medicine for you.

Third tool – Sleep

The third tool that can be used towards fixing or re-setting the circadian rhythm is sleep.

	How many hours of sleep		Minutes in bed before you fall sleep			No. of times waking up for >5 min		
Age	Ideal	Not recommended	Normal	Borderline	Abnormal	Normal	Borderline	Abnormal
0-3 months	14-17	<11 or >19	0-30 min	30-45 min	>45 min	Normal to wake up a few times		
4-11 months	12-15	<10 or >18	0-30 min	30-45 min	>45 min	Normal to wake up a few times		
1-2 years	11-14	<9 or >17	0-30 min	30-45 min	>45 min	1	2-3	>4
3-5 years	10-13	<8 or >16	0-30 min	30-45 min	>45 min	1	2-3	>4
6-13 years	9-11	<7 or >15	0-30 min	30-45 min	>45 min	1	2-3	>4
14-17 years	8-10	<7 or >13	0-30 min	30-45 min	>45 min	1	2	>3
18-25 years	7-9	<6 or >11	0-30 min	30-45 min	>45 min	1	2-3	>4
26-64 years	7-9	<6 or >10	0-30 min	30-45 min	>45 min	1	2-3	>4
>65 years	7-8	<6 or >10	0-30 min	30-60 min	>60 min	2	3	>4

The table above is a comprehensive summary of sleep patterns that you should know as per your age group. The recommended sleep is well displayed here, which means infants 0-3 months of age need 14 to 17 hours of sleep. So if they sleep less than 11 hours or more than 19 hours, they only go on to show some abnormalities which is not recommended. Also, if such infants take more than 45 minutes to sleep after being put to bed, such a factor may also be considered an abnormal pattern.

Similarly, in the bracket of above 18 years and below 65 years of age, the amount of sleep could range between 7 to 9 hours, In case you are in this bracket and tend to sleep less than 6 hours or more than 9 hours then once again, you are bound to disturb your body clock, inviting diseases in the long run. Also, if your sleep pattern after hitting the bed is delayed for about 45 to 60 minutes, it means there is a certain disturbance in your body clock. Another abnormal activity is your need to get up 3-4 times at night, whereas simply getting up once is considered normal.

So it is crucial you keep a check on abnormal patterns of sleep and maintain a balanced body rhythm. Let us take an example of a shift worker who sleeps during the day in order to be able to work well at night. It is not unusual for such a worker to keep shifting the sleep pattern often. This is most unfortunate as it is well researched fact that shift workers suffer from more diseases than those who do not work at night or the normal population. This way they are more prone to obesity, stroke, cancer, diabetes heart disease and metabolic syndromes.

Sleep ←——→ Shift worker [15]

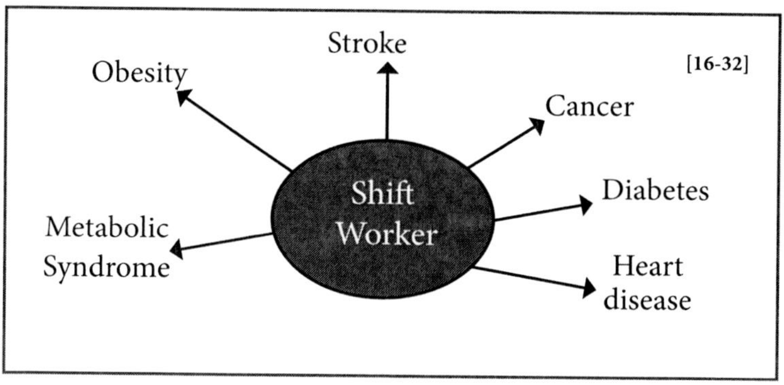

Therefore, disturbance in sleep disturbs your circadian rhythm.

Ancestral sleep patterns

The sleep table provided in the previous pages is based upon how our ancestors used to sleep. Our ancestral societal living patterns did not permit light beyond sunset, may be only 50 lux of fire light beyond evening time. This way they slept at sunset and were awake with sunrise. Such patterns also lead to extending their life-span. This is because it is a proven fact that those who have disturbed sleep patterns die early. Also, people who have disturbed sleep tend to be more obese. Another interesting fact about such sleep disorders is the food choices such people make. This connection with bad sleep with bad kind of fast food or unhealthy food such as chocolates, noodles, cold-drinks, chips etc. On the contrary, if you have a good sleep and then you feel hungry, you are more likely to choose good food such as fruits, vegetables, nuts or seeds. All this means once you start taking care of your sleep and start to follow the ancestral sleep patterns to a certain extent, your circadian rhythm will start to reset and your body will become healthy again.

Ancestral Sleep [33]

Sleep Disturbance $\propto$ Mortality [34]

Sleep ⟶ Obesity Connection [35]

Sleep ⟶ Food Choice Connection [36]

Light ⟷ Body Clock[37]

Later Circadian Timing [38]

Circadian Triangle

Now that I have introduced you to the factor of earthing in order to bring back your circadian rhythm, I would also like you to know the other two factors of the circadian triangle that help regain the circadian rhythm or balance your body clock.

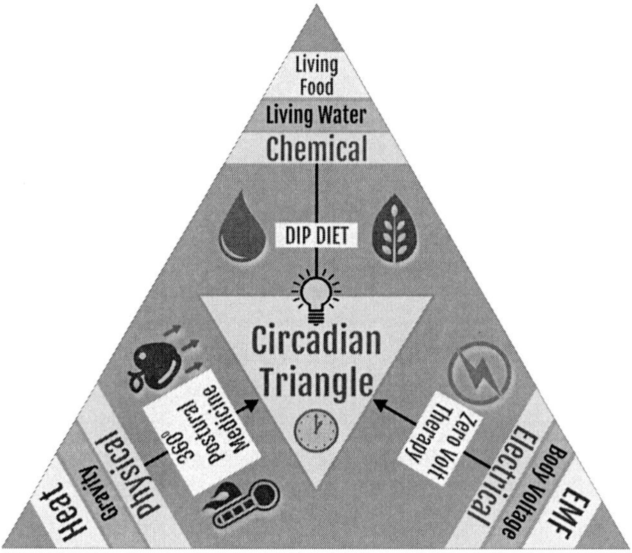

The second factor being the choice of healthy food what we call as the DIP diet that brings back the chemical balance of the body. Those who have gone through my *'Medical Nutritional Training Programme'* will understand this better. The third factor that helps the body clock balance is the heat and gravity. Those who have taken our training on *'Emergency and Pain Management'* through Sridhar University, understand the importance of gravity and heat in order to maintain good health. Hot water immersion and Ayurvedic Panchkarma are used to utilise the power of heat and the force of gravity in correcting the body clock. I encourage you to read my book "360^0 Postural Medicine" to understand the practical application of heat & force of gravity in reversing a disease and maintaining physical & mental well being.

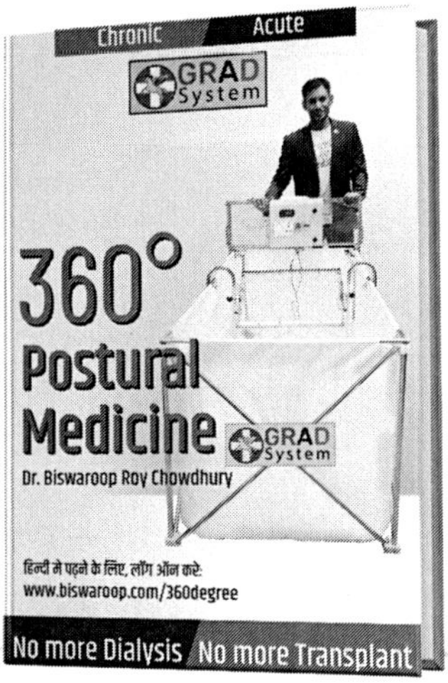

References:

1. *K. P. Wright, Jr. et al., "Entrainment of the Human Circadian Clock to the Natural Light-Dark Cycle," Current Biology 23, no. 16 (2013): 1554–58.*

2. *M. Boubekri, et al., "Impact of Windows and Daylight Exposure on Overall Health and Sleep Quality of Office Workers: A Case-Control Pilot Study," Journal of Clinical Sleep Medicine 10, no. 6 (2014): 603–11.*

3. *J. A. Evans et al., "Dim Nighttime Illumination Alters Photoperiodic Responses of Hamsters through the Intergeniculate Leaflet and Other Photic Pathways" Neuroscience 202 (2012): 300–308*

4. *J. A. Evans et al., "Dim Nighttime Illumination Alters Photoperiodic Responses of Hamsters through the Intergeniculate Leaflet and Other Photic Pathways" Neuroscience 202 (2012): 300–308*

5. C. Cajochen et al., "Evening Exposure to a Light-Emitting Diodes (LED)-Backlit Computer Screen Affects Circadian Physiology and Cognitive Performance," Journal of Applied Physioliology 110, no. 5 (2011): 1432–38

6. R. E. Fargason et al., "Correcting Delayed Circadian Phase with Bright Light Therapy Predicts Improvement in ADHD Symptoms: A Pilot Study," Journal of Psychiatric Research 91 (2017): 105–10.

7. K. A. Stokkan et al., "Entrainment of the Circadian Clock in the Liver by Feeding," Science 291 (2001) 490–93.

8. M. P. St-Onge, et al., "Meal Timing and Frequency: Implications for Cardiovascular Disease Prevention: A Scientific Statement from the American Heart Association," Circulation 135, no. 9 (2017): e96–e121

9. M. Hatori et al., "Time-Restricted Feeding without Reducing Caloric Intake Pre-vents Metabolic Diseases in Mice Fed a High-Fat Diet," Cell Metabolism 15, no. 6 (2012): 848–60.

10. A. Chaix et al., "Time-Restricted Feeding Is a Preventative and Therapeutic Intervention against Diverse Nutritional Challenges," Cell Metabolism 20, no. 6 (2014): 991–1005.

11. A. Zarrinpar et al., "Diet and Feeding Pattern Affect the Diurnal Dynamics of the Gut Microbiome," Cell Metabolism 20, no. 6 (2014): 1006–17.

12. M. Garaulet et al., "Timing of Food Intake Predicts Weight Loss Effectiveness," International Journal of Obesity 37, no. 4 (2013): 604–11.

13. T. Moro et al., "Effects of Eight Weeks of Time-Restricted Feeding (16/8) on Basal Metabolism, Maximal Strength, Body Composition, Inflammation, and Cardiovascular Risk Factors in Resistance-Trained Males," Journal of Translational Medicine 14 (2016): 290.

14. J. Rothschild et al., "Time-Restricted Feeding and Risk of Metabolic Disease: A Review of Human and Animal Studies," Nutrition Reviews 72, no. 5 (2014): 308–18.

15. T. Roenneberg et al., "Epidemiology of the Human Circadian Clock," Sleep Medicine Reviews 11, no. 6 (2007): 429–38.

16. *T. Roenneberg et al., "Epidemiology of the Human Circadian Clock," Sleep Medicine Reviews 11, no. 6 (2007): 429–38.*

17. *D. L. Brown et al., "Rotating Night Shift Work and the Risk of Ischemic Stroke," American Journal of Epidemiology 169, no. 11 (2009): 1370–77.*

18. *M. Conlon, N. Lightfoot, and N. Kreiger, "Rotating Shift Work and Risk of Prostate Cancer," Epidemiology 18, no. 1 (2007): 182–83.*

19. *S. Davis, D. K. Mirick, and R. G. Stevens, "Night Shift Work, Light at Night, and Risk of Breast Cancer," Journal of the National Cancer Institute 93, no. 20 (2001): 1557–62.*

20. *C. Hublin et al., "Shift-Work and Cardiovascular Disease: A Population-Based 22-Year Follow-Up Study," European Journal of Epidemiology 25, no. 5 (2010): 315–23.*

21. *B. Karlsson, A. Knutsson, and B. Lindahl, "Is There an Association between Shift Work and Having a Metabolic Syndrome? Results from a Population Based Study of 27,485 people," Occupational & Environmental Medicine 58, no. 11 (2001): 747–52.*

22. *T. A. Lahti et al., "Night-Time Work Predisposes to Non-Hodgkin Lymphoma," International Journal of Cancer 123, no. 9 (2008): 2148–51.*

23. *S. P. Megdal et al., "Night Work and Breast Cancer Risk: A Systematic Review and Meta-Analysis," European Journal of Cancer 41, no. 13 (2005): 2023–32.*

24. *F. A. Scheer et al., "Adverse Metabolic and Cardiovascular Consequences of Circadian Misalignment," Proceedings of the National Academy of Sciences of the United States of America 106, no. 11 (2009), 4453–58.*

25. *E. S. Schernhammer et al., "Night-Shift Work and Risk of Colorectal Cancer in the Nurses' Health Study," Journal of the National Cancer Institute 95, no. 11 (2003): 825–28.*

26. *E. S. Schernhammer et al., "Rotating Night Shifts and Risk of Breast Cancer in Women Participating in the Nurses' Health Study," Journal of the National Cancer Institute 93, no. 20 (2001): 1563–68.*

27. S. Sookoian et al., *"Effects of Rotating Shift Work on Biomarkers of Metabolic Syndrome and Inflammation," Journal of Internal Medicine 261, no. 3 (2007): 285–92.*

28. *A. N. Viswanathan, S. E. Hankinson, and E. S. Schernhammer, "Night Shift Work and the Risk of Endometrial Cancer," Cancer Research 67 no. 21 (2007): 10618–22.*

29. *E. S. Soteriades et al., "Obesity and Cardiovascular Disease Risk Factors in Firefighters: A Prospective Cohort Study," Obesity Research 13, no. 10 (2005): 1756–63.*

30. *E. S. Soteriades et al., "Cardiovascular Disease in US Firefighters: A Systematic Review," Cardiology in Review 19, no. 4 (2011): 202–15.*

31. *K. Straif et al., "Carcinogenicity of Shift-Work, Painting, and Fire-Fighting," Lancet Oncology 8, no. 12 (2007): 1065–66.*

32. *C. J. Morris, D. Aeschbach, and F. A. Scheer, "Circadian System, Sleep, and Endocrinology," Molecular and Cellular Endocrinology 349, no. 1 (2012): 91–104.*

33. *H. O. de la Iglesia et al., "Ancestral Sleep," Current Biology 26, no. 7 (2016): R271– 72.*

34. *D. F. Kripke et al., "Mortality Associated with Sleep Duration and Insomnia," Archives of General Psychiatry 59, no. 2 (2002): 131–36.*

35. *S. E. Anderson et al., "Self-Regulation and Household Routines at Age Three and Obesity at Age Eleven: Longitudinal Analysis of the UK Millennium Cohort Study," International Journal of Obesity 41, no. 10 (2017): 1459–66.*

36. *S. M. Greer, A. N. Goldstein, and M. P. Walker, "The Impact of Sleep Deprivation on Food Desire in the Human Brain," Nature Communications 4 (2013): article no. 2259.*

37. *F. Damiola et al., "Restricted Feeding Uncouples Circadian Oscillators in Peripheral Tissues from the Central Pacemaker in the Suprachiasmatic Nucleus," Genes and Development 14 (2000): 2950–61.*

38. *A. W. McHill et al., "Later Circadian Timing of Food Intake Is Associated with Increased Body Fat," American Journal of Clinical Nutrition 106, no. 6 (2017): 1213–19.*

CHAPTER -5

Circadian Dining Table

(Adapted from Dr BRC's lecture in Cure@72hrs program)

We have gone through the importance of body clock balancing in the previous chapters, based on the circadian rhythm along with the timing of food intake. The timing of your food intake, which seems like a small thing, is actually one of the most important factors around food, because of this you will be able to get rid yourself of from any kind of disease. A well-known adage says that 'your diet is a bank account and good food choices are your good investments'. However, let us keep aside your diet and your food-choices for the time being and concentrate on just the timing of your food intake in this chapter. Your best diets and good food choices can bring in diseases if you are busy eating anytime you feel hungry. So let us look into a unique formula in this chapter that I have devised for your good health – it is called the **Circadian Dining Table.**

Circadian Dining Table

For a better understanding, you can take three plates of food – one for breakfast, one for lunch and the third for dinner – as pointed in the picture on the next page.

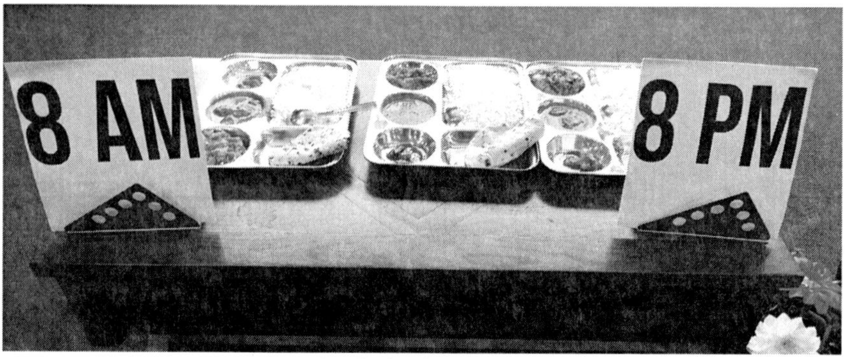

Standard Indian Food-Plate

These are three standard Indian plates with chapattis, seasonal vegetables, pulses and some rice. Biggest quantity of food on the breakfast plate followed by a little less on the lunch plate and the least food on the dinner plate - assuming that the breakfast time is 8:00 am followed by lunch in the afternoon and dinner to be consumed by 8:00 pm. This is what I call the circadian dining table. Now let us assume that after consuming these plates in a 12-hour window, a person accounts for 150mg/dl blood sugar. This means his body is in a healthy state.

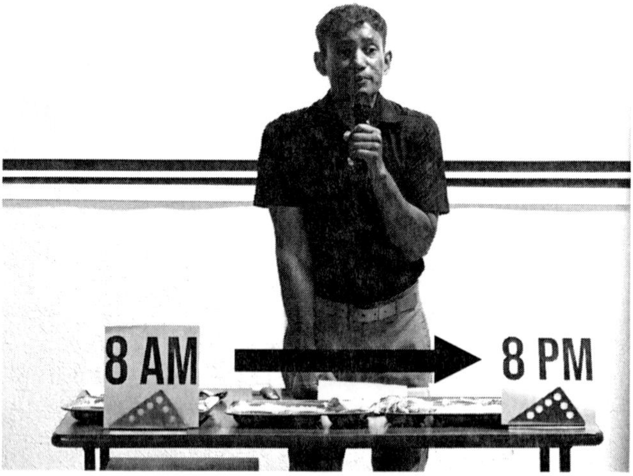

12 hours' time window between 8AM to 8PM

Now if we wish to make him a sugar patient, all we need to change is to re-distribute the quantity of his food intake in the same 12-hour window. So, the order of the food plates goes this way – least amount of food at breakfast, then more quantity of food at lunch and the maximum quantity of food at night.

I have not increased the food on the plates but only changed the order in which the same quantity of food to be consumed by the same person but at different times. In other words, the person will now have the least food for breakfast and most at the dinner time. By just shuffling the breakfast & dinner the blood sugar is expected to rise by say 50mg/dl. But in this case hypothetically it will be about 200mg/dl. This is the same person eating in the same 12-hour window between 8:00 am and 8:00 pm. However, in this case, the same amount of food plates are consumed at different times of the day.

What happened that this change happens in blood sugar? What was the reason of blood sugar increase? The simple reason is the natural clock of pancreas in a human body being most active at around 8:00 am. Also, the least active time of pancreas is near and beyond 8:00 pm. Now if we eat least amount of food at 8:00 am, when the insulin secretion in the body and pancreatic digestion is at its peak, and eat most at the time of least insulin production, then the reverse results are expected.

Noticeably, people are seen skipping their breakfast or else having very little for breakfast whereas, it is strongly recommended to have most food at breakfast time. This is when the insulin production is at its best. In case your body produces insulin at this time and you underutilize it or do not choose to utilize it at all, your body clock automatically starts getting disturbed.

Disturbing the blood sugar further

So now I have successfully tampered with sugar levels of a healthy person by shuffling the food plates on the dining table thereby changing the quantity of food intake. But if I have to make a permanent sugar patient, I will tamper with the time factor of this healthy person.

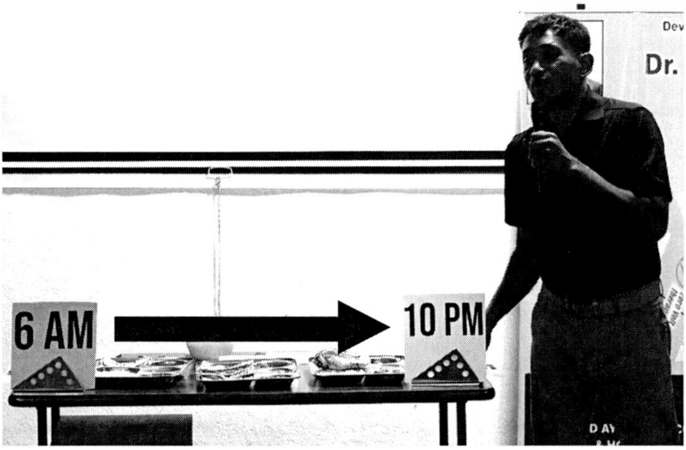

Time window between 6AM to 10PM (14hrs time window)

This time I have simply increased the window of time for the food intake. However, I have not brought any changes in food quantity. It is the same quantity of food that he was consuming. But now the same three meals he is taking at 6:00 am instead of 8:00 am and the final dinner at 10:00 pm instead of 8:00 pm – by this time his pancreas is fast asleep. So now you should be having a clear idea that food is not responsible for his diabetes but the larger window of food intake timing may make him diabetic. Doctors will never tell you to reduce the time window of your food intake. They will suggest blood sugar lowering drugs and insulin. Relevant research papers supporting the above explanations are given on the next page:

Circadian rhythms and pancreas physiology: A review

Front. Endocrinol., 10 August 2022 Sec. Diabetes: Molecular Mechanisms
Volume 13 - 2022 | https://doi.org/10.3389/fendo.2022.920261

Christopher J. Morris, Jessica N. Yang, Joanna I. Garcia, Samantha Myers, Isadora Bozzi, Wei Wang, Orfeu M. Buxton, Steven A. Shea, and Frank A. J. L. Scheer

Effect of meal timing and glycaemic index on glucose control and insulin secretion in healthy volunteers

Published online by Cambridge University Press: 16 December 2011

Authors Linda M. Morgan, Jiang-Wen Shi, Shelagh M. Hampton and Gary Frost

Endogenous Circadian system and circadian misalignment impact glucose tolerance via separate mechanisms in humans

Medical Institute, University of Texas Southwestern Medical Center, Dallas, TX, and approved March 20, 2015 (received for review October 1, 2014) April 13, 2015 112 (17) E2225-E2234 on and Gary Frost

High Caloric intake at breakfast vs. dinner differentially influences weight loss of overweight and obese women ***First published: 20 March 2013 https://doi.org/10.1002/oby.20460***
Authors: *Daniela Jakubowicz, Julio Wainstein, Oren Froy*

Effect of a late supper on digestion and the absorption of dietary carbohydrates in the following morning ***Journal of Physiological Anthropology volume 32, Article number: 9 (2013)***
Authors: *Yukie Tsuchida, Sawa Hata & Yoshiaki Sone*

What can make the blood sugar more erratic?

By skipping breakfast on continuous basis, one should expect the unexpected, his blood sugar may further rise.

In other words, if I stop him to have his breakfast in the morning, his pancreas is expected to slowly stop producing the digestive insulin in his body during morning hours. A point to be remembered here is whenever pancreas will not produce insulin at the right time, which is morning 8:00 am, there are bound to be other biological changes in hormones throughout the body. So, if I have to create a permanent insulin patient, I don't have to give him more food to eat, but decrease his food intake by making him skip his breakfast. Breakfast skipping is expected to disturb the homeostasis of blood sugar. So, point is not only what you are eating or how much, but whether you are eating at the right time or not. If you do skip sometimes due to some reasons, it's okay however you must not skip breakfast on a continuous basis. Following are the research papers supporting the above logic.

Breakfast skipping and the risk of Type 2 Diabetes: a meta-analysis of observational plan. ***Published online by Cambridge University Press: 17 February 2015***
Authors: *Huashan Bi, Yong Gan, Chen Yang, Yawen Chen, Xinyue Tong and Zuxun Lu*

Skipping Breakfast and Risk of Mortality from Cancer, Circulatory Diseases and All Causes: Findings from the Japan Collaborative Cohort Study ***Yonago Acta Med. 2016 Mar*** ***Authors:*** *Yukie Tsuchida, Sawa Hata & Yoshiaki Sone*

Making of a cancer patient

There are many studies that indicate major harm to the body if you skip breakfast. Extending the same example to create cancer patient, let me again change the time frame of the food intake. Instead of starting the breakfast at 8:00 am in the morning, start eating breakfast at 10:00 pm every night and eat the same quantity of food all night intermittently until 6:00 am in the morning.

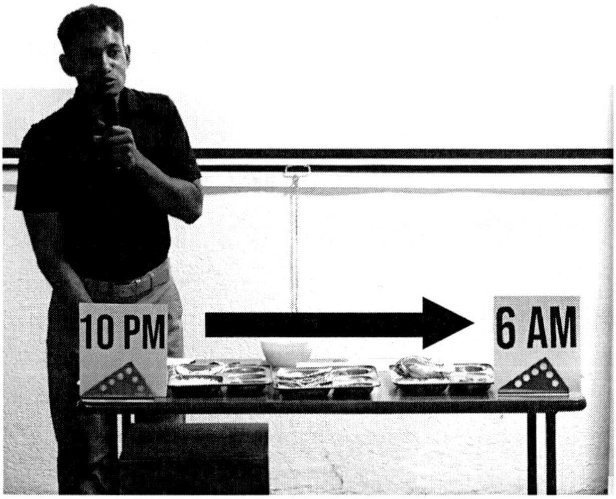

Time window between 10PM - 6AM (night-shift work hours)

The quantity of food is still the same – except the timing of food intake. There are many people who work in late night shifts. They are all set to eat through the night. People who are night watchmen/soldiers or marine workers or else from other professions that involve working in the nights who are bound to eat at the night time. Most of the night workers have higher mortality rates and suffer from innumerable and unwanted diseases. This is because once you start eating at nights, your body may start losing its body clock. So, eating during the night time as a habit, can consequently produce cancer in the body.

Just like a soldier on the border accepts that he can get a bullet anytime, you must accept this too that if you are choosing a hazardous profession, you are sure to incur imbalance in body clock and hence get into a vicious cycle of diseases. So, you will need to make the right choices about your profession, which is directly related to your lifestyle. There are many who do not even have a professional compulsion to remain awake at night, yet are found eating during the nights due to their faulty lifestyle. It's not necessary that you are eating throughout the night, it can be as simple as late eating until 11 pm – all these habits amount to disturbing your body clock and inviting diseases.

Solution and cure

Until now, I have pointed out how various kinds of diseases are developed in your body, now I will tell you how to cure these diseases.

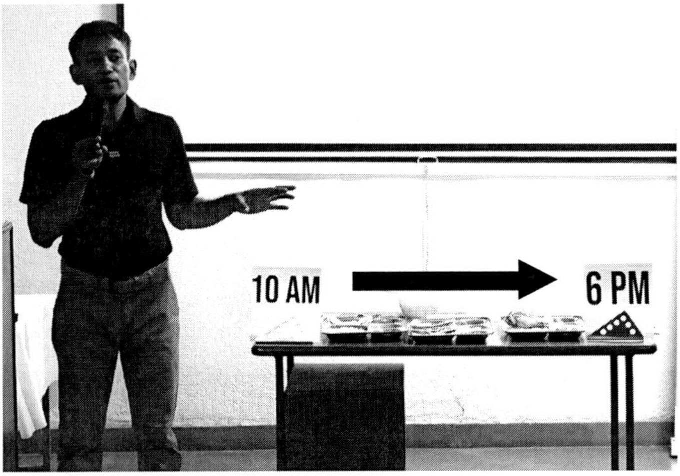

Ideal eating time window between 10AM to 6PM (8 hrs eating window)

The perfect clock timing of any human body is breakfast time that starts from 10:00 am and dinner time that ends by 6:00 pm.

Importantly, your body functions in an amazing manner so that if you eat within the bracket of 10:00 am and 6:00 pm any outgrowth within the body starts getting dissolved. Outgrowths within the body can come in the form of tumors, stones in kidney and gall bladder, fibrosis, fibromyalgia, internal blockages, etc. All this is expected to dissolve slowly if this bracket of eating time is maintained.

This time bracket of eating between 10:00 am and 6:00 pm is also related to obesity. If someone is obese, you just need to make sure he or she eats within this time bracket.

If we seek the reasons for such simple and time restricted cures for such deadly diseases, the answer would be that this kind of research called '**autophagy**' has fetched Nobel Prize four times – not just once. Once the body is starving, the internally outgrown cells that are termed as diseases like tumor or stones but in the real sense nothing but deposits of protein, calcium, potassium, and other kinds of nutrition – will be broken down. Such a process often leads to finishing off the tumors and other internal outgrowths. But the body will only utilize the excess minerals and proteins when you manage your food intake within this time-frame. The time of intake has to be during the day-time, not at night – as pointed earlier. Research papers supporting the above logic are given below:

Obesity, cancer risk, and time-restricted eating

Cancer Metastasis Rev. 2022 Sep;41(3):697-717. doi: 10.1007/s10555-022-10061-3.

Sleep ⟶ Obesity Connection

S. E. Anderson et al., "Self-Regulation and Household Routines at Age Three and Obesity at Age Eleven: Longitudinal Analysis of the UK Millennium Cohort Study,"

International Journal of Obesity 41, no. 10 (2017): 1459–66.

Circadian disruption enhances HSF1 signalling and tumorigenesis in Kras-driven lung cancer ***SCIENCE ADVANCES 28 Sep 2022 Vol 8, Issue 39 DOI: 10.1126/sciadv.abo1123*** ***Authors:*** *MARIE PARIOLLAUD , LARA H. IBRAHIM, EMANUEL IRIZARRY, REBECCA M. MELLO, ALANNA B. CHAN BRIAN J. ALTMAN REUBEN J. SHAW H8977, MICHAEL J. BOLLONG 6, R. LUKE WISEMAN, AND KATJA A. LAMIA*

Time as medicine

Time-restricted eating has major benefits on health and has potential to bring back good health.

You can follow the simple time rule as follows:

1. First 15 days – food intake in 8-hour window only.
2. Next 15 days – food intake in 10-hour window only.
3. There-on, Lifelong - food intake in 12-hour window only.

Time as Medicine
• **8 hrs window of eating (1st 15 days)** • **10 hrs window of eating (next 15 days)** • **12 hrs window of eating (lifelong)**

Expectedly, over a period of one month, most of the people will have gotten over with their maladies, be it tumor kinds of outgrowths or water retention, or stones, or anything else. If you have cleared your system of a specific disease by using 10/8 hours rule, you can increase the window for the rest of your life. In the above slide, the first two (8hrs/10hrs) are applicable for getting your circadian rhythm back in cycle and the proactive way to remain disease-free is where the third (12hrs) is applicable.

Power of circadian clock

As per a particular study that carried out research on 15,000 farmers in Sri Lanka who had taken poison for killing themselves. This poison was nothing but the pesticides that they used on their farms. As per the data collected, among the farmers who consumed pesticides in the evening hours fewer deaths were reported as against those who had taken the same pesticide during the morning hours. This just goes on to prove the power of timing when our body is metabolically more active. During the evening time, the poison could not be processed well in the body towards digestion, whereas in the morning time, the poison was processed immediately. That is the power of circadian clock.

Diurnal variation in probability of death following self-poisoning in Sri Lanka--evidence for chronotoxicity in humans.

Int J Epidemiol. 2012 Dec;41(6):1821-8.doi: 10.1093/ije/dys191. Epub 2012 Nov 23.
Author: Robert Carroll 1, Chris Metcalfe, David Gunnell, Fahim Mohamed, Michael Eddleston

Food

There are factors other than the time factor that impact your body clock either positively or negatively. One of the most important of those factors is Food. Many of the readers must already be following the DIP Diet. In the DIP diet, we take nothing but fruits until 12:00 noon. The reason being, fruits are naturally endowed with more sugar, fructose, carbohydrates, minerals etc. We also know by now that your body's digestive juices too are most productive in the morning hours. This means if you have lots of minerals and vitamins in the morning, your body will start giving you extra energy right from the morning hours. So, make sure you have a stomach - full of fruits intake in the morning.

First step of DIP diet

The DIP diet rule otherwise depends on your body weight multiplied by ten. Suppose your body weight is 70 kgs then multiplying with 10 will give 700. So, make sure you take approximate 700 grams of fruits intake. However, stick to the simple rule of eating the plate of fruit as per your hunger. Remember that you need to have maximum quantity of food in the morning so have fruits and do not keep your stomach empty by skipping breakfast.

DIP Diet
Step -I
Breakfast (till 12 noon) **4 types of fruit** **Weight in kg x 10=__gm**

The Govt. of India conducted a clinical trial of the DIP diet in the year 2018. It clearly states how this DIP diet helps in the control of different diseases, be it thyroid or bones related diseases. The trial reports have been successfully published in various journals as well as on Govt. of India clinical trial registry.

Thus, we must understand that this diet is already proven and established. Anyone who now adopts this diet in their lifestyle for their own benefit will not be experimenting in any way. You can simply help cure all of your illnesses and diseases by using this scientifically proven diet without having to doubt or worry about it.

Relevant links to all journals and references are given ahead:

DIP Diet
Clinical trial of the DIP Diet by All India Institute of Ayurveda (Under Ministry of AYUSH, Govt. of India) *Ctri/2018/12/016654*

DIP Diet
Case Study – Reversal of Type 1 Diabetes Using Plant Based Diet *Journal of the Science of Healing Outcomes, Jan 2021 (Vol 13, No. 50)*

DIP Diet

To Evaluate the Efficacy of Agnikarma and Disciplined and Intelligent Person Diet in Katigata-Sandhivata w.s.r to Lumbar Spondylosis – A Case Report.

Int J Ayu Pharm Chem 2020 Vol. 13 Issue 1

Second step of DIP diet

The second step of DIP diet is what is it that you should focus on having in lunch and dinner. There are two types of plates during lunch time - plate one of lunch time will have four types of raw vegetables as salad. If you multiply your body weight with five, then that should be the ideal quantity (in grams) of raw vegetable intake.

DIP Diet

Step -II

Lunch/Dinner

Plate-1	Plate-2
4 types of raw vegetables	Std. meal

Weight in kg x 5=_ gm

Once you consume the raw vegetables, your body will release a hormone called incretin. This hormones is secreted in the gut region right after our intake of food that helps to stimulate insulin secretion. These secretions are released into the blood stream within minutes of eating in order to regulate the appropriate amount of insulin to be secreted after eating.

Once you have finished eating the plate-1 (raw salad), you can eat your traditional vegetarian food as plate-2, as per your appetite.

Third step of DIP diet

Let us now take a look at the third step of the DIP diet. There are only two things that I request my patients to abstain from when following this step. The first important category to avoid is packaged food. This includes any food item that is produced in a factory such a namkeen packets, bread, or biscuits. The second important category is animal or dairy foods. In this category, the food source is an animal. This includes meat, fish, eggs and chicken. This category also includes all dairy products like cheese, butter, milk or buttermilk etc. So, the third step to follow DIP diet is to avoid the two categories of food that can help reverse your body clock.

DIP Diet	
Step -III	
<u>To Avoid</u> **1. Packed food** **2. Dairy/Animal food**	**<u>To Take</u>** **1. Soaked nuts/Sprouts: your wt(kg)=.. gm** **2. Fruits: Plenty** **3. Sunshine: 40 min**

Remaining connected to earth

Think of traveling to a different time zone while keeping your mobile in flight mode. Say you are flying from India to USA. Upon landing in US your mobile will still show the time in accordance to Indian time zone, from where you started. Only after connecting the mobile to the local internet, the mobile will readjust itself and pick up the local time.

Similarly, your body-clock is set in accordance to Indian time zone from where you started. So, upon landing in place with different time zone, we feel jet lag i.e., feel sleepy the whole day while sleepless at night, for several days. To correct the body-clock, you need to get connected to the earth, i.e., let your skin touch the earth. This you can achieve by walking barefoot on earth (not on concrete) for few minutes. The moment you touch the earth surface, within the first 10 seconds, your body voltage becomes zero, as literally electrons flow from earth to your body. You can also remain in contact with earth via conductive wire as we do in our hospitals, where patients, are grounded for at least 8 to 10 hrs. per day, through a zero-volt bed sheet, in which a copper wire is connected to the earth. This leads to continuous reduction in inflammation resulting in various health benefits as given below:

Zero Volt (Earth) Therapy	
Time	**Effect on body**
10 Seconds	Your body voltage will be zero
20 minutes	Improvement in mood/stress
30-45 minutes	Relief from palpitation
1 hour	Pain relief
1-2 hour	Better sleep
Overnight	Fast wound healing, less stiffness, Parkinson relief, reduction in B.P.
7 days	Reduced B.P. (for diabetes patients)
1 month	Blood disorder reversal

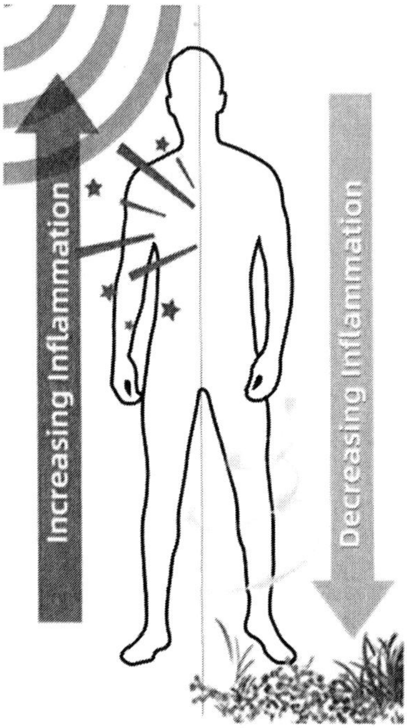

Below are the research paper supporting the above explanations:

One-hour contact with the Earths's surface (grounding) improves inflammation and Blood Flow- A Randomized, Double-Blind, Pilot Study

DOI: 10.4236/health.2015.78119

Author: Gaétan Chevalier, Gregory Melvin & Tiffany Barsotti

The biologic effects of grounding the human body during sleep as measured by cortisol levels and subjective reporting of sleep, pain, and stress

PMID: 15650465 DOI: 10.1089/acm.2004.10.767

Author: Maurice Ghaly & Dale Teplitz

Earthing: Health Implications of Reconnecting the Human Body to the Earth's Surface Electrons

J Environ Public Health. 2012; 2012: 291541

Author: Gaétan Chevalier, Stephen T. Sinatra, James L. Oschman, Karol Sokal, and and Pawel Sokal

The Circadian Chart

Be it cancer, heart disease or kidney failure, to my understanding, the best way to bring back the health is by resetting the body clock. At my hospitals, I try to treat the patients by correcting the 7 checkpoints, as given in the circadian chart (please refer to the back inner cover of the book). Ahead in the book you will find the observational study and success stories of my patients, who followed some of the advices, mentioned in this book. Also go to www.coronakaal.tv to find more than 10,000 video testimonials of the patients who reversed their illnesses by following my advices of making small adjustments in their lifestyle.

CHAPTER -6

First 72 hrs of Correcting the Circadian Clock

By now you know that the rule-4 of the treatment of cancer which is equally effective and necessary in treating and curing all kinds of lifestyle oriented illnesses.

What will happen in the first 72 hrs of correcting the Circadian Clock?

In this section, I share the summary of the observational study done through the collaborative efforts of Dayanand Ayurvedic College, Jalandhar. The study was done on our recently concluded (16th to 19th March 2023) 'Cure@72hrs' program at Dayanand Ayurvedic College, Jalandhar with a total of 50 patients. The key guidelines maintained during the 72 hrs stay of the patients are:

1) Patients were encouraged to sleep in accordance with their age, as per the table given below.

	How many hours of sleep		Minutes in bed before you fall sleep			No. of times waking up for >5 min		
Age	Ideal	Not recommended	Normal	Borderline	Abnormal	Normal	Borderline	Abnormal
0-3 months	14-17	<11 or >19	0-30 min	30-45 min	>45 min	Normal to wake up a few times		
4-11 months	12-15	<10 or >18	0-30 min	30-45 min	>45 min	Normal to wake up a few times		
1-2 years	11-14	<9 or >17	0-30 min	30-45 min	>45 min	1	2-3	>4
3-5 years	10-13	<8 or >16	0-30 min	30-45 min	>45 min	1	2-3	>4
6-13 years	9-11	<7 or >15	0-30 min	30-45 min	>45 min	1	2-3	>4
14-17 years	8-10	<7 or >13	0-30 min	30-45 min	>45 min	1	2	>3
18-25 years	7-9	<6 or >11	0-30 min	30-45 min	>45 min	1	2-3	>4
26-64 years	7-9	<6 or >10	0-30 min	30-45 min	>45 min	1	2-3	>4
>65 years	7-8	<6 or >10	0-30 min	30-60 min	>60 min	2	3	>4

2) We tried to maintain zero voltage of the patients, at least 10 hrs per day. This was achieved by placing a zero-volt bed sheet in their rooms.
3) Food in accordance with the DIP diet was provided during the entire stay.
4) Living water was provided from 3-pot water system during the entire stay. To know more about it, read my book "The Cure for Blood Disorders".
5) To achieve physical balance, based on their symptoms (swelling, pain etc.), patients were given specific therapies like hot water immersion, head down tilt, heat protocol or panchakarma, etc.
6) Patients were encouraged to get at least 10,000 lux of light for more than 30 minutes during the first half of the day and were also asked to avoid the light of more than 50 lux at least 2 hours before sleep.
7) Patients were served food within the bracket of 10 hours i.e. between 9.00 am to 7:00 pm. For a time between 7:00 pm and to next day 9:00 am, they are asked to avoid eating. Drinking water was allowed without any restrictions.
8) Other vitals like blood sugar, blood pressure, body weight, pain intensity, and energy level were collected several times per day during their entire stay in the hospital. Blood sugar sensors were implanted in the arms of 8 diabetes patients.
9) Drugs were tapered in accordance with the improvement of various parameters.

Key Outcomes Of 'Cure@72hrs' Program at Dayanand Ayurvedic College Jalandhar (16th to 19th March 2023)

1. Out of 50 patients, 24 patients were diabetic and 100% of the patients could lower their blood glucose levels without any medicines.
2. 4 patients were taking insulin before joining the cure@72hrs program. 50% were completely free from insulin and remaining 50% could reduce their insulin dosage by half.
3. 12 patients were on antihypertensive drugs, out of them 11 stopped their medicines and were still able to either lower or maintain same BP.
4. Those who were overweight could lower their weight with an average of 2 kgs in three days, with one patient losing more than 5 kgs and one losing 3 kgs.
5. Underweight patients were 5 in number and out of them 2 could gain weight with an average of 1 kg, one patient witnessed no change while one lost weight further.
6. 66% (i.e., 33 out of total 50) of the participants had noticeable improvement in their energy levels, 28% could maintain their energy levels to same level while only 3 patients felt low energy.
7. Out of 50 participants, 28 were having some or the other kind of pain 12 persons i.e., 43% were either completely free from pain or reduced the pain remarkably, 12 patients had no significant improvement.
8. 83% of 11 patients with constipated bowel felt complete evacuation, 3 were having no significant improvement.
9. Out of 2 patients who were complaining of loose stools before joining the program, one had improvement and his bowel movement was normal. 4 out of 50 had incomplete evacuation.

10. 12 patients were facing disturbed sleep or insomnia and out them 9 i.e., 75% had better sleep from the very first day of their joining the camp.
11. 75% of 12 patients who complained of swelling could reduce their swelling to more than 75%. 17% did not notice any change and 1 patient complained of increased swelling.
12. 18 Patients were given LLHWI (Lower Leg Hot Water Immersion). Out of the 14 i.e., 77.77% could lower their BP within half an hour by an average of 20 systolic and 10 diastolic without any medicine.

Noticeable Points:

1) Participant Snehlata's sugar reading reduced from 307mg/dl to 136mg/dl within 48 hrs without any medicines.
2) Participant Rekha Meshram was insulin free within 48 hrs. She was taking 20 units before coming to Cure@72 hrs program.
3) Bakshish Singh's BP reduced from 170/100 mmHg to 120/70 mmHg within 48 hrs without any medicinal intervention.
4) Inderjit Type 1 patient could reduce his insulin dose from 46U to 19U within 48hrs of Cure@72hrs Program.
5) Bhawna Talwar's weight reduced from 110 kg to 107.5 kg within 72 hrs of the camp
6) Harish Khimraj Gala reduced 2 kg weight, BP reduced from 160/100mmHg to 140/90mmHg, Sugar reduced from 223mg/dl to 131mg/dl while being medicine free.
7) Deepak Verekar was suffering from excessive sleep disorder and was sleeping more than 12 hrs at night, his sleep normalized to 7 hrs within 10 hrs of sleeping on Zero Volt Bedsheet.

8) Md Mukhtar's frequency of urination from 5 times at night reduced to 2 times within 48 hrs of joining the camp.
9) Nitin Garg's high BP 160/110mmHg reduced to 110/90 within 20 minutes of LLHWI (lower leg hot water immersion).
10. Navjot Singh could reduce his weight by 5 kgs (85 kg to 80 kg) within 72 hrs of the camp.
11. Bhartee Devi was complaining of weight loss problem, her weight increased from 47 kg to 49 kg during 3 days of the camp.

Refer to the 'Cure@72hrs' poster given at the end of the book.

CHAPTER -7

Success Stories

1

Aggressive Angiomyxoma

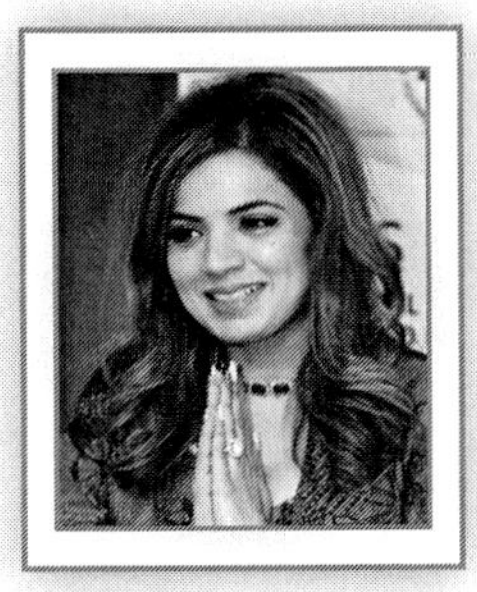

Vidhika Batra, age 44 years / female, resides in Delhi.

She was diagnosed with 'aggressive angiomyxoma' on May 15, 2015. Just before the diagnosis she had irregular periods, spotting and excessive bleeding. Doctors advised her to go for CT scan of the lower abdomen and that was the first time aggressive angiomyxoma was diagnosed and chemotherapy was started at Max Hospital, Saket, New Delhi.

Following were Vidhika Batra's parameters before starting DIP Diet:

Medication taken: Nil

Physical Symptoms/Discomforts: Irregular periods, excessive bleeding and spotting.

She came into contact with us in January 2021 and started the DIP Diet.

The present status after starting the therapy:

Medications: None

Physical Symptoms/ Discomforts: Nil

Special Remark: Vidhika Batra having reversed her cancer, now runs her own HIIMS Premier Hospital at Gurugram, Haryana. Under her guidance many patients have recovered from some major illnesses.

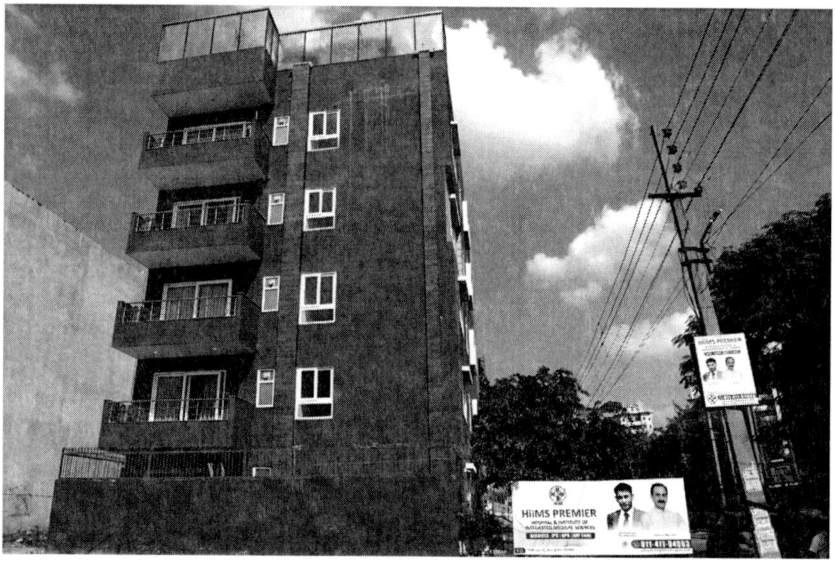

Note: *To access the diagnostic reports and video testimonial of the patient, please go to:* [*www.biswaroop.com/rtm*](www.biswaroop.com/rtm)

2

Liver Hemangioma & Kidney Cyst

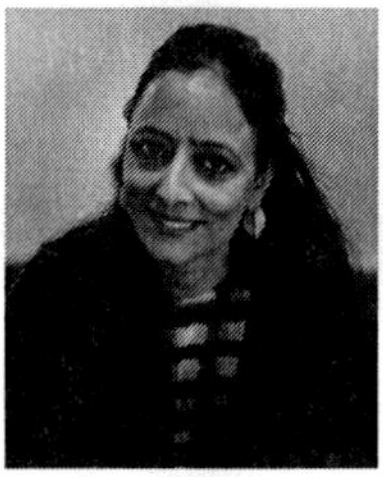

Dr Namita Gupta, MBBS, MD, age 52 years/female, resides in New Delhi.

Dr Namita was diagnosed with Hemangioma Liver and Kidney Cyst on 13 August 2018. She went for a regular check-up and underwent an ultrasound. That was the first time her Liver Hemangioma and Kidney Cyst were diagnosed. She never visited any doctor after that

Following were Dr Namita's parameters before starting DIP Diet:

Medication taken: Nil

Physical Symptoms /Discomforts: Nil

She came into our contact in 2021, by that time she had already started the raw diet.

The present status after starting the therapy:

Medications: Nil

Physical Symptoms/ Discomforts: Nil

Special Remark: She has completely reversed both the problems. She now actively treats patients through DIP diet and Living Water Therapy and is working with Dr. BRC Team

Note: *To access the diagnostic reports and video testimonial of the patient, please go to: www.biswaroop.com/rtm*

3

Multiple Tumors in Lower Spine

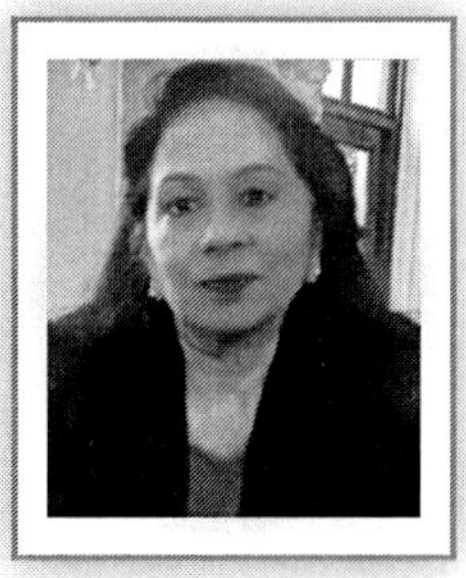

Simmi Handa, age 58 years / female, resides in New Delhi.

She was diagnosed with multiple tumors in lower spine in 2002. Just before the diagnosis she experienced severe pain in her back and body. Doctors advised her to go for an MRI, PET scan and that was the first-time multiple tumors in lower spine were diagnosed at Rajiv Gandhi Hospital, Rohini, New Delhi. Chemotherapy was advised but she never underwent any allopathic treatment.

Following were Simmi Handa's parameters before she started raw diet:

Medication taken: Calcium supplements

Physical Symptoms /Discomforts: Severe pain in back and body

The present status after starting the therapy:

Medications: Nil

Physical Symptoms/ Discomforts: Nil

Special Remark: Nothing less than a miracle from Medical Science point of view, Simmi Handa (Pharmacist), with severe osteoporosis of (-6), bedridden for almost one year, walking with the help of clutches, followed by the diagnosis of cancer; is now a marathon runner, a full-time proponent of the DIP Diet and a part of W.I.S.E Team.

Note: *To access the diagnostic reports and video testimonial of the patient, please go to: www.biswaroop.com/rtm*

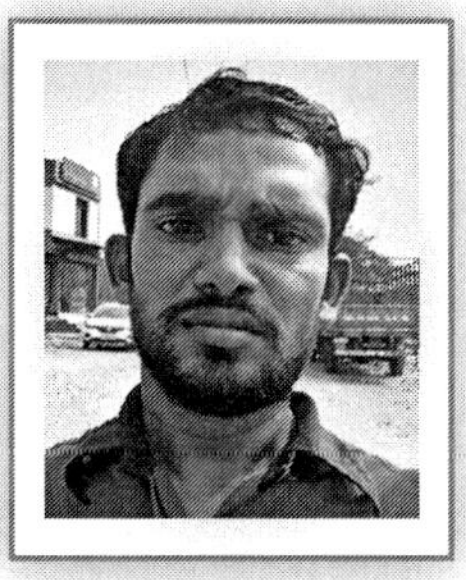

4

Brain Tumor

Gajendra Kashyap, age 32 years / male, resides in Bilaspur, Chhattisgarh

He was diagnosed with a brain tumor in December 2022. Before the diagnosis he had giddiness, uneasiness and depression. Doctor advised him to go for CT scan and that was the first time a brain tumor was diagnosed and surgery was advised by the doctors at Apollo Hospital. Instead, he directly contacted Dr Biswaroop Roy Chowdhury's Team through Virtual OPD.

Following were Gajendra Kashyap's parameters before starting DIP Diet:

Medication taken: Nil

Physical Symptoms /Discomforts: Giddiness, uneasiness, depression.

He came into our contact in January 2022 through Virtual OPD and started the DIP Diet.

The present status (as on 24 March 2023) after starting the DIP Diet and Postural Therapy:

Medications: Nil

Physical Symptoms/ Discomforts: Nil

Special Remark: He started feeling good within 15 days of diet & fully recovered within 3 months. He is now encouraging and helping his thalassemic nephew follow the Living Water Therapy to make him free from blood transfusions.

***Note:** To access the diagnostic reports and video testimonial of the patient, please go to: www.biswaroop.com/rtm*

5

Non-Hodgkin's Lymphoma

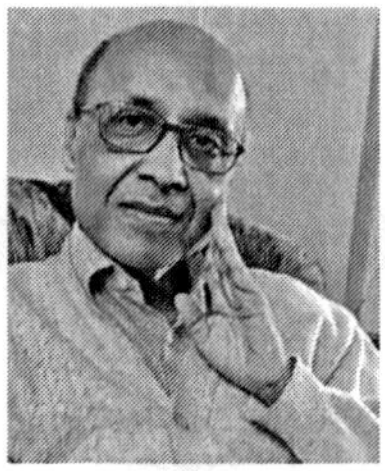

Arvind Jain, age 58 years / male, resides in Ballygunge, Kolkata.

He was diagnosed with Non-Hodgkin's lymphoma in July 2021. Just before the diagnosis he had a lump around his neck. Doctor advised him to go for PET-CT followed by biopsy and that was the time, Non-Hodgkin's lymphoma was diagnosed. Just after diagnosis he directly contacted Dr Biswaroop Roy Chowdhury through Virtual OPD.

Following were Arvind Jain's parameters before starting DIP Diet:

Medication taken: Nil

Physical Symptoms /Discomforts: Lump around the neck

He came into our contact on 14 July 2021 through Virtual OPD and started the DIP Diet.

The present status after starting the therapy:

Medications: Nil

Physical Symptoms/ Discomforts: Nil

Special Remark: Arvind Jain was advised to undergo immediate surgery as according to the doctors non-Hodgkin's lymphoma was a fast spreading cancer. But not only it stopped growing within six months of following the DIP Diet and Postural therapies, it regressed from 3 cm to 2 cm. Even allopathic doctors were surprised at this development. At present the lump has disappeared physically but can be felt very lightly when touched by hand.

***Note:** To access the diagnostic reports and video testimonial of the patient, please go to: www.biswaroop.com/rtm*

6

Cervix Cancer

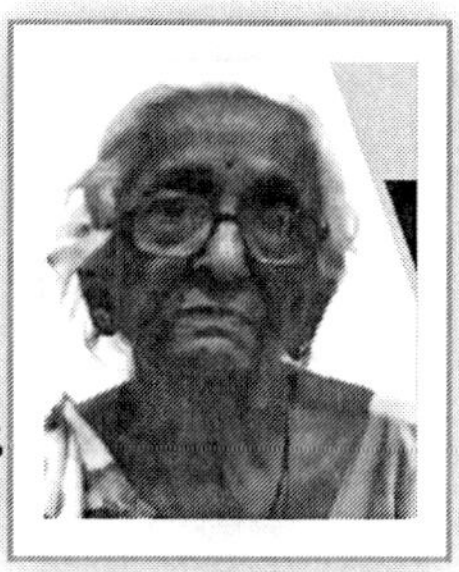

Tara Ben Patel, age 73 years / female, resides in Jaipur, Rajasthan.

She was diagnosed with cervix cancer in the year 2020. Just before the diagnosis, she was passing out blood in urine. Doctors advised her to go for PET scan followed by biopsy and that was the first-time cervix cancer was diagnosed and was advised to undergo surgical removal of the uterus at Manipal Hospital, Jaipur, Rajasthan.

Following were Tara Ben Patel's parameters before starting DIP Diet:

Medication taken: Tab Pregabid-nt OD, Tab Dexona 2mg OD, Tab Emset 4mg OD, Tab A to Z gold OD

Tab Pan d BD, Saline nasal spray, Betaloc 50 OD, Torsemide & Spironolactone half tablet OD

Pantocid DSR OD, Alprax plus

Physical Symptoms /Discomforts: Low pitch in voice, body fatigue and weakness post 100-meter walk, numbness in feet, nose blockage while breathing.

She came into our contact on 5 April 2021 through Virtual OPD and started the DIP Diet.

The present status after starting the therapy:

Medications: Nil

Physical Symptoms/ Discomforts: Nil

Special Remark: Doctors told her family that she will not be able to survive more than 1 year. It has now been more than 3 years, and she is healthy without any medication. Even doctors are amazed.

Note: *To access the diagnostic reports and video testimonial of the patient, please go to: www.biswaroop.com/rtm*

7

Suspected Lung Cancer

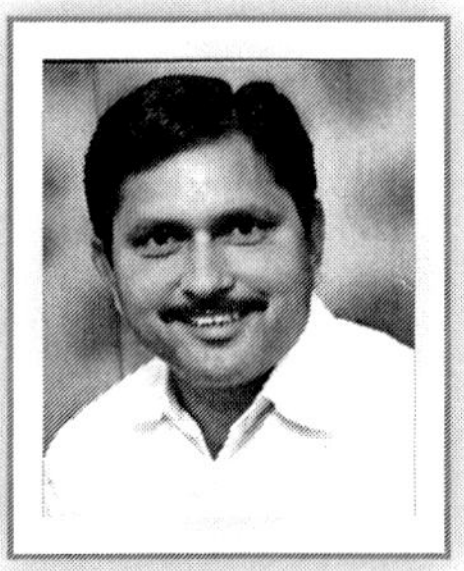

Ajit Singh Yadav, age 49 years / male, resides in Gurugram, Haryana.

He had severe coughing, breathlessness and blood in cough. He visited doctors who suspected lung cancer and was advised to undergo PET scan by doctors at Fortis hospital, but he avoided any test and directly contacted Dr Biswaroop Roy Chowdhury.

Following were Ajit Singh Yadav's parameters before starting DIP Diet:

Medication taken: Nil

Physical Symptoms /Discomforts: Severe coughing, blood in cough, breathlessness

He came into our contact on 17 July 2022 through Virtual OPD and started the DIP Diet and Postural Therapies.

The present status after starting the therapy:

Medications: Nil

Physical Symptoms/ Discomforts: Nil

Special Remark: He lost his wife 2 years ago because of cancer treatment, so having witnessed first-hand bitter experience of cancer treatment, when he was suspected with lung cancer with severe symptoms, he followed the DIP Diet protocol and today he is fit & fine without any medicine, allopathic treatment or any other therapy.

***Note:** To access the diagnostic reports and video testimonial of the patient, please go to: www.biswaroop.com/rtm*

8

Cervix Cancer

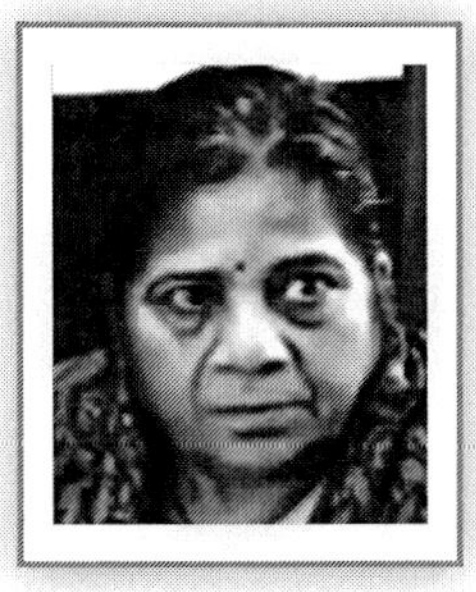

Seema, age 65 years / female, resides in New Delhi.

She was diagnosed with cervix cancer in November 2022. Just before the diagnosis she had severe pain in lower abdomen, back pain, knee pain, & breathlessness. Doctor advised her to go for MRI and PET scan and that was the time cervix cancer was diagnosed and she was advised surgical removal of uterus at Safdarjung Hospital and Lady Hardinge Medical College, New Delhi.

Following were Seema's parameters before starting DIP Diet:

Medical Condition: Cervix Cancer

Physical Symptoms /Discomforts: Pain in lower abdomen, severe back pain, knees' pain, breathlessness.

Medication taken: Nil

They came into our contact on 7 November 2022 and took DIP Diet treatment at HIIMS Hospital Derabassi.

The present status after starting the therapy:

Physical Symptoms/ Discomforts: Nil

Medications: Nil

Special Remark: When she came to know about her cancer she was scared to death as she lost her husband earlier due to several treatment procedures in the hospital. She now, after getting cured, looks forward to a healthy long life.

***Note:** To access the diagnostic reports and video testimonial of the patient, please go to: www.biswaroop.com/rtm*

9

Brain Tumor

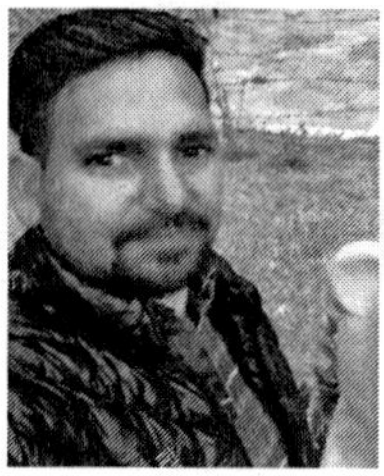

Balwinder Singh, age 35 years / male, resides in Rajpura, Punjab.

He was diagnosed with Brain Tumor in December 2020. Just before the diagnosis he had headaches and 70 to 80% blurred eye vision. Doctor advised him to go for CT scan and that was the first-time brain tumor was diagnosed and he was advised surgery and radiotherapy at PGI Patiala.

Following were the parameters before starting DIP Diet:

Medication taken: Nil

Physical Symptoms / Discomforts: Headache, Eye vision blurred 70-80%

He came into our contact on 8 September 2022 through Virtual OPD and started the DIP Diet and Postural Therapies.

The present status after starting the therapy:

Medications: Nil

Physical Symptoms/ Discomforts: Eye vision blurred at 70%

Special Remark: Tumor has regressed considerably as per PET scan reports after 9 months of following DIP diet and therapies.

Note: PET scan is unreliable test.

Note: *To access the diagnostic reports and video testimonial of the patient, please go to: www.biswaroop.com/rtm*

10

Non-Small Cell Lung Cancer

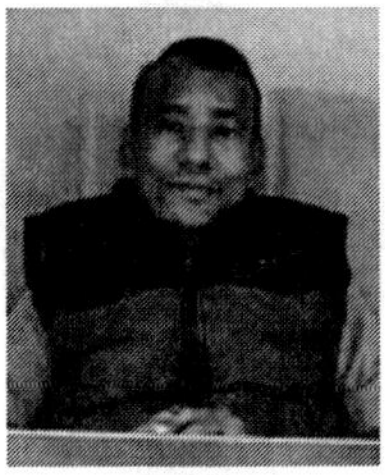

Kishor Silwal, age 44 years / male, resides in Chitwan, Kathmandu.

He was diagnosed with non-small cell lung cancer stage 4 in February 2022. Just before the diagnosis he had severe pain in spine & weakness. Doctors advised him to go for CT scan & biopsy and that was the first time when non-small cell lung cancer stage 4 was diagnosed and conventional treatment was started at Rajeev Gandhi Hospital, Delhi.

Following were Kishor Silwal's parameters before starting DIP Diet:

Medication taken: Zoldonat injection, Calcium tablets, Alectinib 600 mg twice a day, medicine for constipation.

Physical Symptoms /Discomforts: Severe spine pain, physically very weak, unable to walk, no appetite.

He came into our contact in October 2022 through Virtual OPD and started the DIP Diet protocol.

The present status after starting the therapy:

Medications: Alectinib 600 mg / once a day

Physical Symptoms/ Discomforts: Nil

Special Remark: Before starting the DIP Diet, he could barely sit or walk properly. Today he has resumed office work, performs his routine chores and plays sports in the playground actively.

***Note:** To access the diagnostic reports and video testimonial of the patient, please go to: www.biswaroop.com/rtm*

11

Lump on Neck

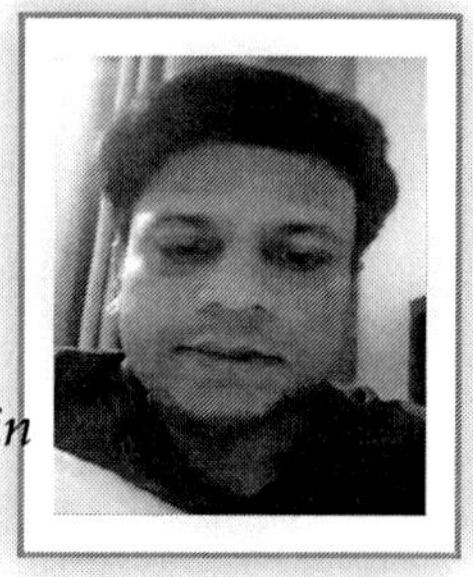

Deepak Kumar Sahu, age 38 years / male, resides in Kanpur, Uttar Pradesh.

He felt a lump on his neck while taking a head massage in November 2022. He directly contacted Dr Biswaroop Roy Chowdhury for Virtual OPD.

Following were Deepak Kumar Sahu's parameters before starting DIP Diet:

Medication taken: Nil

Physical Symptoms /Discomforts: Pain in lump while touching.

He came into our contact on 10 November 2022 through Virtual OPD and started the DIP Diet.

The present status after starting DIP Diet and Postural Therapy:

Medications: Nil

Physical Symptoms/ Discomforts: Nil

Special Remark: Lump on his neck has reduced by 50% within one month and is hardly visible.

Note: *To access the diagnostic reports and video testimonial of the patient, please go to: www.biswaroop.com/rtm*

12

Renal Cell Carcinoma

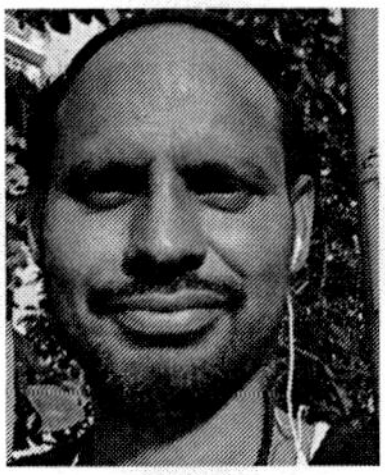

Vikas Gupta, age 40 years / male, resides in Ghaziabad, Uttar Pradesh.

He was diagnosed with renal cell carcinoma in November 2022. Just before the diagnosis, he had severe pain on front left side and back. He was admitted to the hospital because of dengue and was diagnosed with renal cell carcinoma after doctors advised him to go for ultrasound, MRI, PET scan at B L Kapoor Hospital, New Delhi. He was advised chemotherapy upon diagnosis.

Following were Vikas Gupta's parameters before starting DIP Diet:

Medication taken: Tablet Thyroxine 50 mcg, Tab Cabozantinib 40 mg once a day, Injection Denosumab 120 mg in 28 days & Inj. Opdyta in 15 days for 2 months.

Physical Symptoms /Discomforts: Severe back pain & pain in left side of the abdomen.

He came into our contact through Virtual OPD on 12 January 2023 and started the DIP Diet and Postural Therapy.

Present status after starting the therapy:

Medications: Tablet Thyroxine 25 mcg

Physical Symptoms/ Discomforts: Nil

Special Remark: While losing extra weight, his skin is shining and glowing with health.

Note: *To access the diagnostic reports and video testimonial of the patient, please go to: www.biswaroop.com/rtm*

13

Uterus and Ovarian Cancer

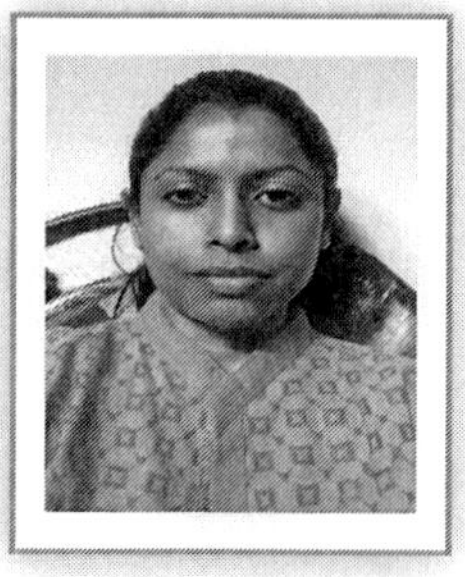

Soma Dey, age 32 years / female, resides in Tezpur, Assam.

She was diagnosed with ovarian cysts after she went to visit a gynecologist for her abdominal pain. Cysts were removed through 3 major surgeries. Upon biopsy of the removed cysts, uterus and ovarian cancer was diagnosed and she was advised for surgical removal of the ovaries and uterus at Gogoi Nursing Home, Tezpur.

Following were Soma Dey's parameters before starting DIP Diet:

Medication taken: Ayurvedic medicines

Physical Symptoms /Discomforts: Weakness, occasional abdominal pain, laziness.

She came into our contact on 15 March 2022 through Virtual OPD and started the DIP Diet.

The present status after starting the therapy:

Medications: Nil

Physical Symptoms/ Discomforts: Nil

Special Remark: After a harrowing physical and mental trauma of 3 major cyst removal surgeries, she has recovered completely

Note: *To access the diagnostic reports and video testimonial of the patient, please go to: www.biswaroop.com/rtm*

14

Left Breast - Infiltrating Duct Carcinoma

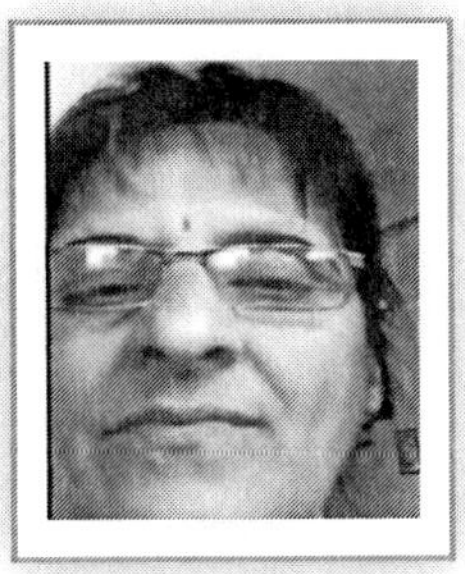

Sumita Roy, age 50 years / female, resides in Raipur, Chhattisgarh.

She had high BP for the last 10 years. She was diagnosed with left breast - infiltrating duct carcinoma in January 2023. Just before the diagnosis, she had difficulty in breathing, heaviness and pain in the breast while walking or getting up after sitting. Doctors advised to go for ultrasound followed by FNAC and that was the first time when left breast - infiltrating duct carcinoma was diagnosed and surgery was advised at AIIMS, Raipur.

Following were Sumita Roy's parameters before starting DIP Diet:

Medication taken: Concor (5 mg)

Physical Symptoms /Discomforts: Breathlessness, heaviness and pain in chest while getting up or walking, dizziness, knee pain, high BP, lump in left breast.

She came into our contact on 25 January 2023 through Virtual OPD and started the DIP Diet.

The present status after starting the therapy:

Medications: Nil

Physical Symptoms/ Discomforts: Nil, lump size reduced.

Special Remark: BP normal, lump size reduced within 2 months of starting the DIP Diet and Postural Therapies.

Note: *To access the diagnostic reports and video testimonial of the patient, please go to:* *www.biswaroop.com/rtm*

15

Lung Cancer

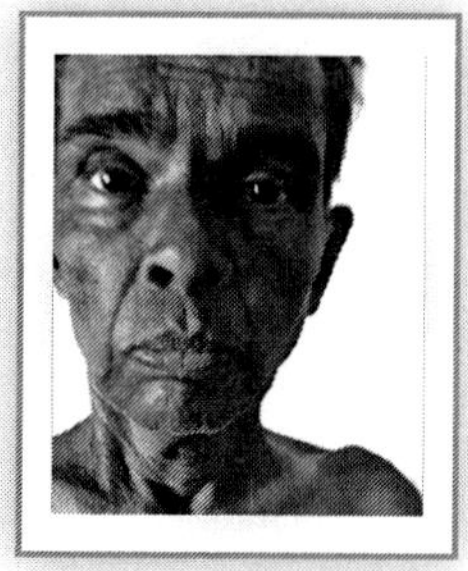

Rameshwar Lal Dudi, age 73 years / male, resides in Bangalore, Karnataka.

He was diagnosed with lung cancer in August 2021. He accidently fell & suffered hairline fracture in ribs, CT-scan revealed dense lesion on his lung. Doctors advised to go for FNAC and non-small cell lung carcinoma was diagnosed at Bikaner, AIR - Bangalore. He immediately contacted us for treatment.

Following were Rameshwar Lal Dudi's parameters before starting DIP Diet:

Medical Condition: Non-Small Cell Lung Carcinoma

Co- morbidities: Diabetes, heart Disease, thyroid

Medication taken: Thyroxine, Glimepiride tablets I. P. Pregabalin & Methylcobalamin Capsules, (Nervisol - PM), Methylcobalamin, Alpha Lipoic Acid, Vitamin D3, Pyridoxine Hydrochloride & Folic Acid Tablets, Rabeprazole Sodium (EC) & Levosulpiride (SR) Capsules (Robrox-L), Calcium Carbonate, Calcitriol, Vitamin K27, Mecobalamin, Magnesium, Boron & Zinc Softgel Capsules, (Zenon- CT) - 01 Capsule every alternate day after dinner (multivitamin).

Physical Symptoms /Discomforts: Itching on body.

He came into our contact on 13 August 2021 through Virtual OPD and started the DIP Diet.

The present status after starting the therapy:

Medications: Thyroxine

Physical Symptoms/ Discomforts: Slight itching still persists.

Special Remark: Freedom from medicine and health reversal.

Note: *To access the diagnostic reports and video testimonial of the patient, please go to: www.biswaroop.com/rtm*

16

Squamous Cell Carcinoma

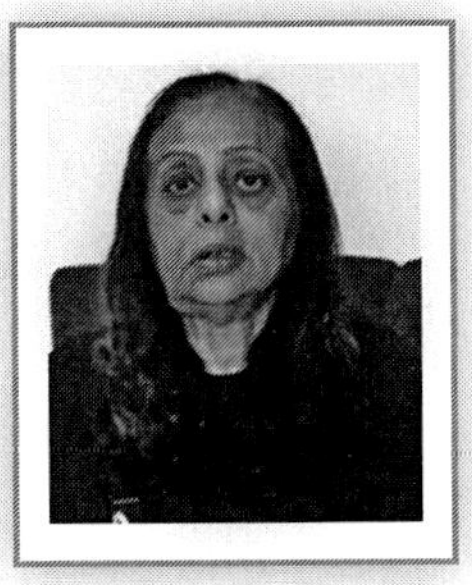

Kanta Shamdasani, age 63 years / female, resides in Andheri West, Mumbai.

She was diagnosed with oral cancer (squamous cell carcinoma) in November 2022. Just before the diagnosis she had gone for a tooth extraction. The Doctor showed her a mass in her mouth and advised her to go for a biopsy and that was when she was diagnosed with squamous cell carcinoma and was advised chemotherapy at Hinduja Hospital.

Following were Kanta Shamdasani's parameters before starting DIP Diet:

Medical Condition: Squamous Cell Carcinoma, diabetes

Medication taken: Glide, Glyciphage, Vitamins Becosules and RockBon

Physical Symptoms /Discomforts: Nil

She came into our contact on 16 January 2023 and started the DIP Diet.

The present status after starting the therapy:

Medications: Nil

Physical Symptoms/ Discomforts: Nil

Special Remark: This is a typical case of indolent cells that was harmless until disturbed either through diagnostic procedures or through chemo, radio or surgery. Additionally, she also got freedom from diabetes medicine.

***Note:** To access the diagnostic reports and video testimonial of the patient, please go to: www.biswaroop.com/rtm*

17

Hodgkin's Lymphoma

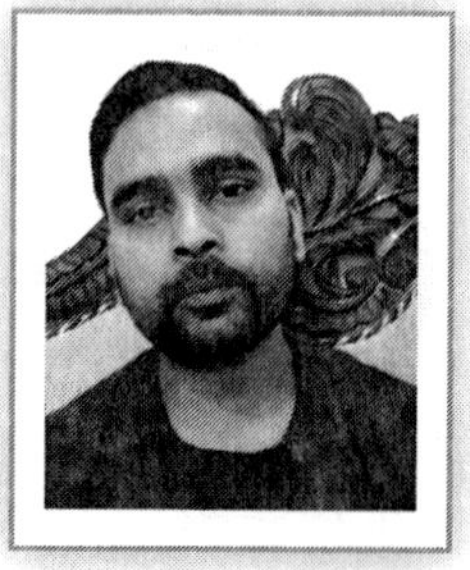

Ravi Kumar Mondal age 25 years/male, resides in Ghazipur, Uttar Pradesh.

Ravi was diagnosed with Hodgkin's Lymphoma on 16 January 2023. Just before the diagnosis, he felt a hard lump around his neck so he underwent a surgical removal of the lump on 18 December 2022. On conducting the biopsy of the removed lump, it was found to be cancerous. By that time two more lumps developed, so doctors advised FNAC and both the lumps were also found to be cancerous. That was the first time Hodgkin's Lymphoma was diagnosed and 12 cycles of chemotherapy was advised. But he never visited the doctor again and took admission in HIIMS Premier Gurugram.

Following were Ravi Mondal's parameters before starting DIP Diet:

Medication taken: Nil

Physical Symptoms /Discomforts: Hard Lumps around Neck and Chin

He came into our contact on 15 February 2023 through HIIMS Gurugram and started the DIP Diet.

The present status after starting the therapy

Medications: Homeopathy Medicines

Physical Symptoms/ Discomforts: Nil

Special Remark: The lumps have softened, as earlier they were hard. No increase in size or number of lumps since then.

Note: *To access the diagnostic reports and video testimonial of the patient, please go to: www.biswaroop.com/rtm*

18

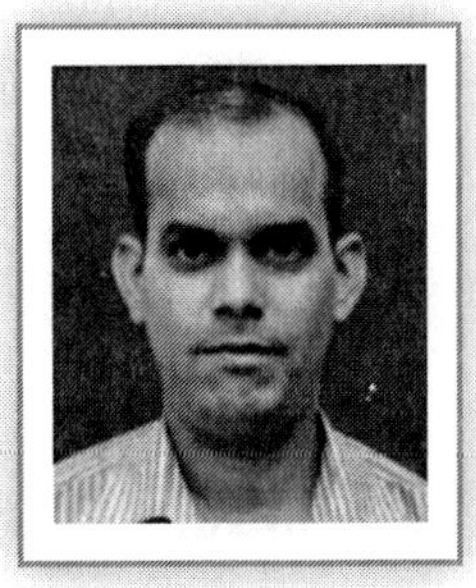

Brain Tumor

Anil Kumar, age 51 years / male, resides in Noida, UP.

He was diagnosed with a brain tumor in 2014. Just before the diagnosis he had giddiness, weakness & recurring headaches. Doctor advised him to go for MRI/ CT scan and that was the first time a brain tumor was diagnosed and a surgery was advised to remove the tumor by the doctors at Safdarjung & AIIMS Hospital, New Delhi. Instead, he directly contacted Dr Biswaroop Roy Chowdhury through Virtual OPD.

Following were Anil Kumar's parameters before starting DIP Diet:

Medication taken: Nil

Physical Symptoms /Discomforts: Giddiness, weakness, headaches.

He came into our contact in 2014 through Virtual OPD and started the DIP Diet.

The present status after starting the therapy:

Medications: Nil

Physical Symptoms/ Discomforts: Nil

Special Remark: After 14 years Anil Kumar is absolutely healthy.

Note: *To access the diagnostic reports and video testimonial of the patient, please go to: www.biswaroop.com/rtm*

19

Thyroid Papillary Carcinoma

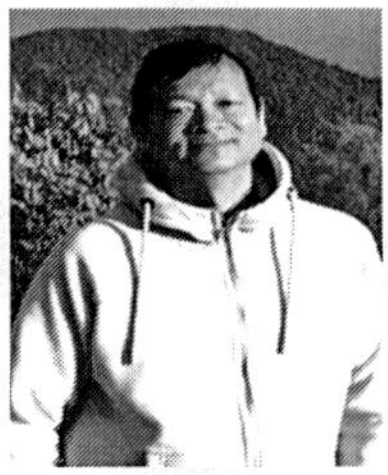

Sanad Piya, age 52 years / male, resides in Chitvan, Kathmandu, Nepal.

He was diagnosed with thyroid papillary carcinoma in June 2021. Just before the diagnosis he had a sudden weight loss of around 11 kgs, so he went to the doctor and underwent several tests. Doctors advised him to go for a biopsy and that was the first time thyroid papillary carcinoma was diagnosed and was advised surgery in Medicity, Nepal and B L Kapoor Hospital, New Delhi but he never visited the hospitals after that and decided to follow our DIP Diet treatment protocol.

Following were Sanad Piya's parameters before starting DIP Diet:

Medication taken: Thyronorm, Sartel 40

Physical Symptoms /Discomforts: Lack of energy, pain in hip bone, weakness, dizziness, 11 kg weight loss.

He contacted one of his good friends, who is a huge follower of Dr Biswaroop Roy Chowdhury in August 2021 and started the DIP Diet.

The present status after starting the therapy:

Medications: Nil

Physical Symptoms/ Discomforts: Nil

Special Remark: Within 11 months of the DIP Diet, FNAC reports for cancer diagnosis came out negative.

Note: FNAC reports are unreliable and we don't recommend it.

Note: *To access the diagnostic reports and video testimonial of the patient, please go to: www.biswaroop.com/rtm*

20

Suspected Urinary Bladder Cancer

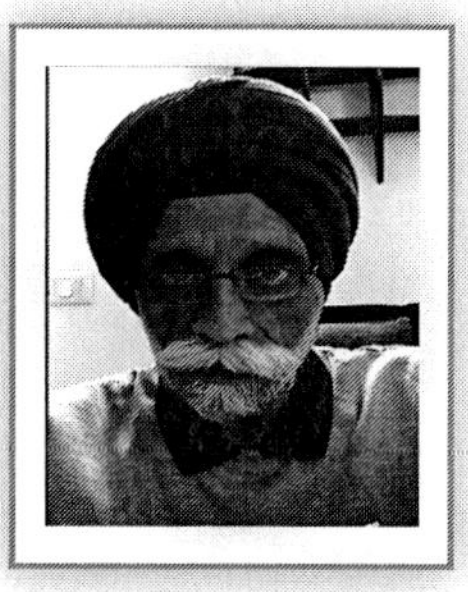

Trilok Singh age 75 years/male, resides in Jalandhar Punjab.

Trilok Singh was suspected of having Urinary Bladder Cancer in December 2022. Since long time he had constipation, acidity and gas and was consuming medicines for the same. In December 2022 he observed blood in urine quite frequently and went for a check up. Upon endoscopy, a tumor was detected and doctors suspected Urinary Bladder cancer and advised surgery. He immediately contacted Dr Biswaroop Roy Chowdhury through online Virtual OPD.

Following were Trilok Singh's parameters before starting DIP Diet:

Medication taken: Nebistar 2.5mg, Ayurvedic tablet, PAN D

Physical Symptoms/Discomforts: Blood in urine, BP,constipation, acidity, gas

On 14th February 2023 he contacted us through Virtual OPD and started the DIP Diet and Postural Therapies.

The present status after starting the therapy

Medications: Nil

Physical Symptoms/ Discomforts: blood in urine after long intervals.

Special Remark : Freedom from medicines and long term suffering from digestive problems of constipation, acidity, gas and BP. He feels light and energetic and is relieved that the bleeding in urine has decreased tremendously.

Note: *To access the diagnostic reports and video testimonial of the patient, please go to: www.biswaroop.com/rtm*

LINCOLN UNIVERSITY COLLEGE

3 Months Online Certification

on

Advance Nutrition Therapy

from

Lincoln University College, Malaysia

Overview: From common cold to Cancer, from headache to heart attack, you can be your own healer. This training comes with a unique tool kit packed with 28 ingredients, the right combination of it can work as a medicine for more than 60 kinds of common illnesses. This training will empower you with skills to heal and will make you realize that your home is the best place to reclaim your health.

Duration: 3 Months

Content:

- Diagnosis of Lifestyle Illness
- Diagnosis of Infectious Diseases
- Food –Medicine Interaction
- Mechanism of Medicine in Body
- Mechanism of Food in Body
- When the Food is Medicine
- When Medicine is Poison
- Common Kitchen Herbs and their Medicinal Usages
- Timeline of Recovery of Common Illnesses
- Food Calculation for Overall Nutrition
  Plants V/S Animal Food

Take-Home Material :

- Hospital in a Box
- Game of Life Chart
- Snake Ladder Nutrition Game
- Reference Book

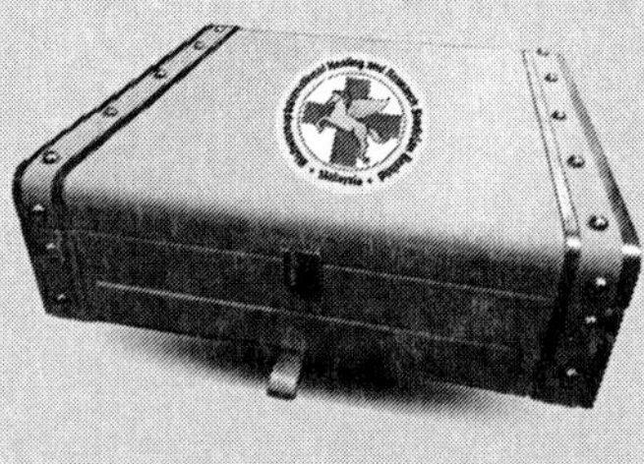

Course Fee: **INR 21,000/- (including GST + Courier)**

Mode of Training: **Online/ viva (oral examination) through a video call**

To register go to www.biswaroop.com/mn

CALL US : +91-9312286540 MAIL US: biswaroop@biswaroop.com

Let every morning be the Hunza Morning

If you have decided to pick only one of my suggestions for the sake of your health, then take this suggestion :

Stop consuming tea specially, morning tea. The early morning tea makes the inner lining of your intestinal wall acidic, as after a long night of fasting your stomach is empty and craving for food. An acidic stomach on a regular basis is the single biggest cause of all kind of inflammatory and lifestyle diseases including arthritis, Diabetes etc.

How to stop craving of tea ⟶ Switch to Hunza Tea

Hunza Civilization: Hunza people are the Indians living at extreme northwest of India in Hindu Kush range. They are known to be one of the world's healthiest civilizations, often living up to the age of 110 years.

How to prepare Hunza Tea (serves four):

Ingredients:

- 12 Mint leaves(Pudina)
- 8 Basil Leaves(Tulsi)
- 4 Green cardamom (Elaichi)
- 2 gm Cinnamon (Dalchini)
- 20 gm Ginger (Adrak)
- 20 gm Jaggery (Gur)

Instructions:

- Take 4 cups of water in a tea pan
- Add all ingredients, simmer it for 10mins
- Add a dash of lemon juice and serve hot or cold

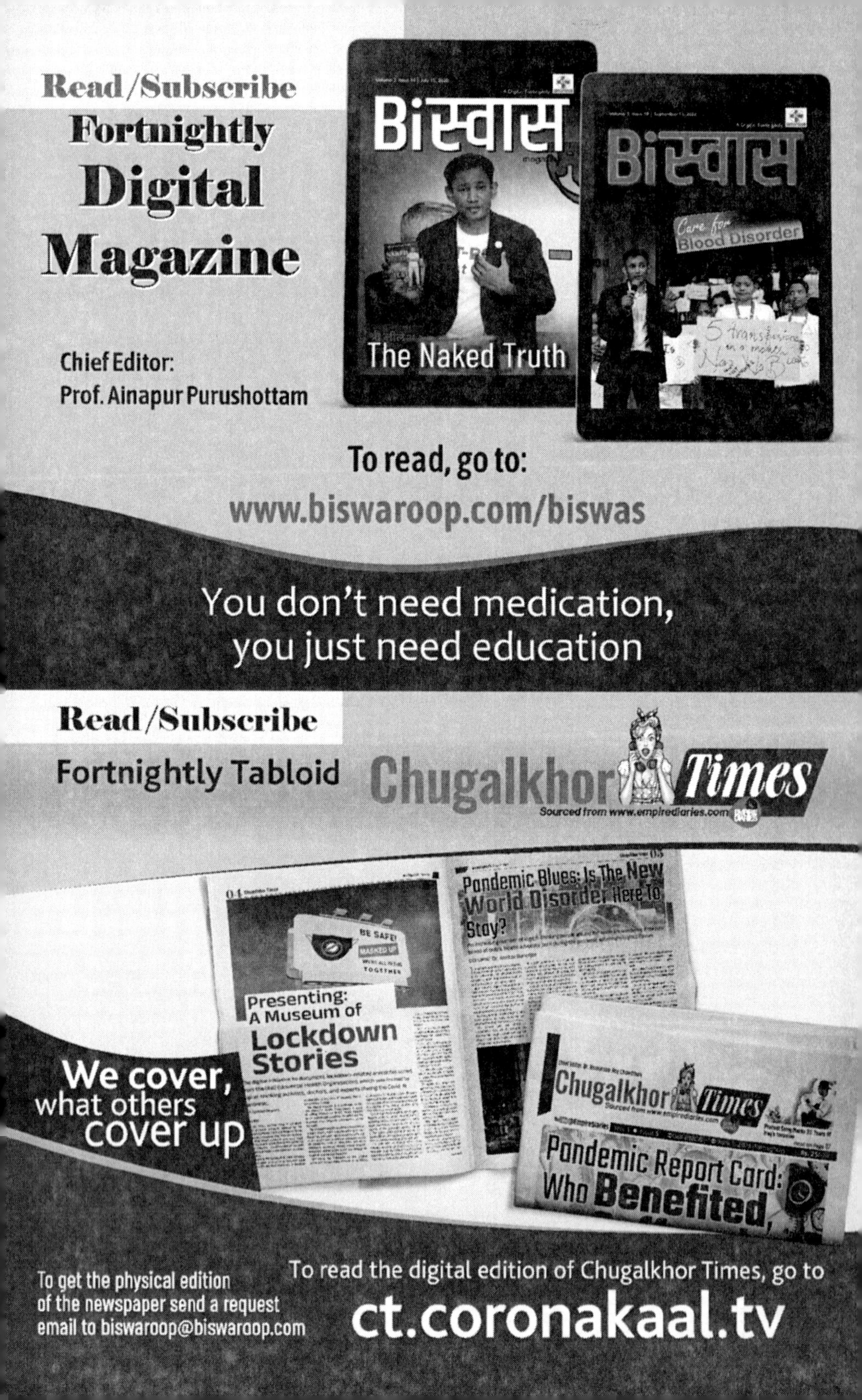
Read/Subscribe
Fortnightly
Digital
Magazine
Chief Editor:
Prof. Ainapur Purushottam
Biस्वास
The Naked Truth
Biस्वास
Care for Blood Disorder
To read, go to:
www.biswaroop.com/biswas
You don't need medication,
you just need education
Read/Subscribe
Fortnightly Tabloid
Chugalkhor Times
Sourced from www.empirediaries.com
Pandemic Blues: Is The New World Disorder Here To Stay?
BE SAFE!
MASKED UP
Presenting:
A Museum of
Lockdown
Stories
We cover,
what others
cover up
Chugalkhor Times
Pandemic Report Card:
Who Benefited,
To get the physical edition
of the newspaper send a request
email to biswaroop@biswaroop.com
To read the digital edition of Chugalkhor Times, go to
ct.coronakaal.tv

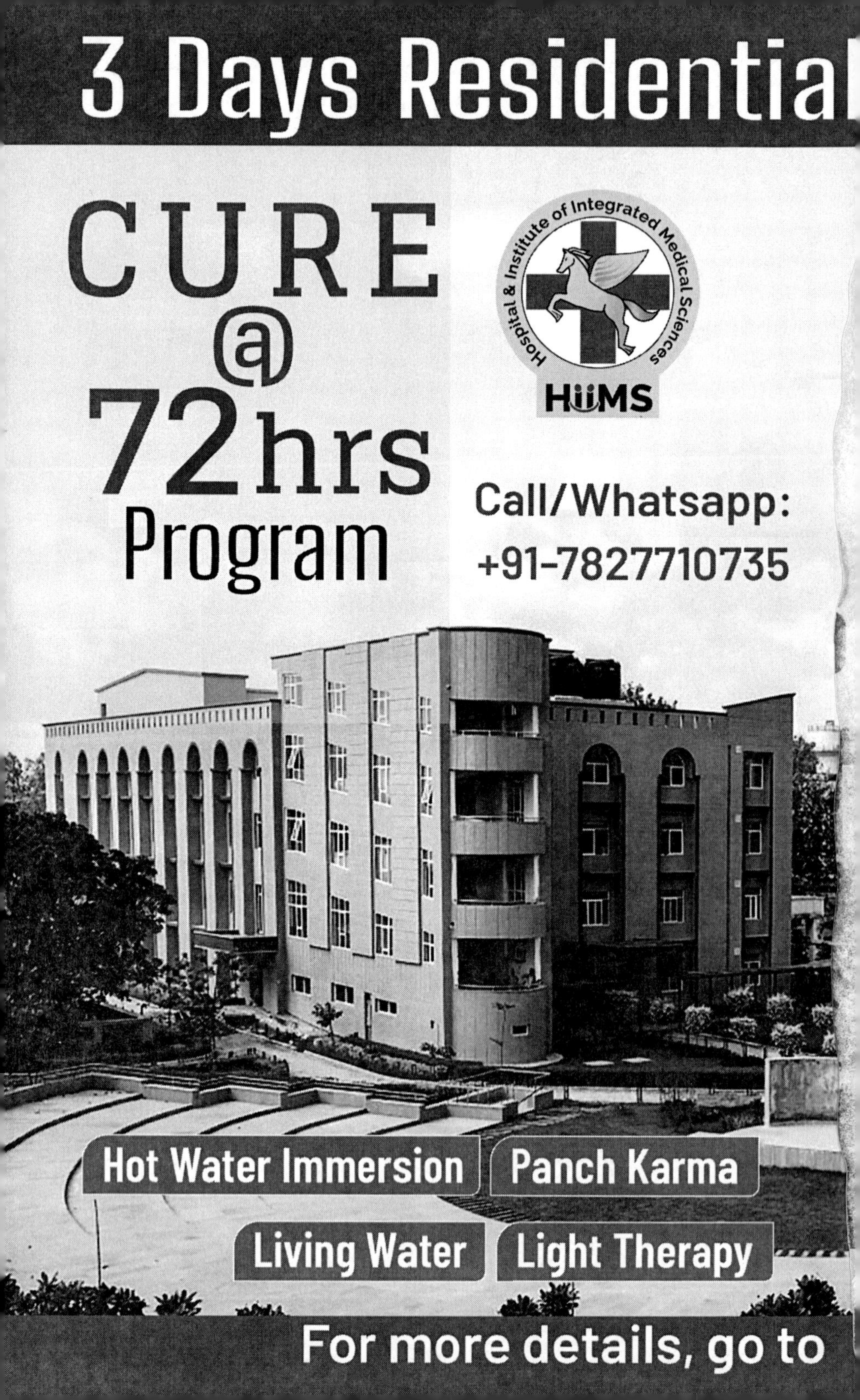
3 Days Residential
CURE @ 72hrs Program
Hospital & Institute of Integrated Medical Sciences
HiiMS
Call/Whatsapp:
+91-7827710735
Hot Water Immersion
Panch Karma
Living Water
Light Therapy
For more details, go to

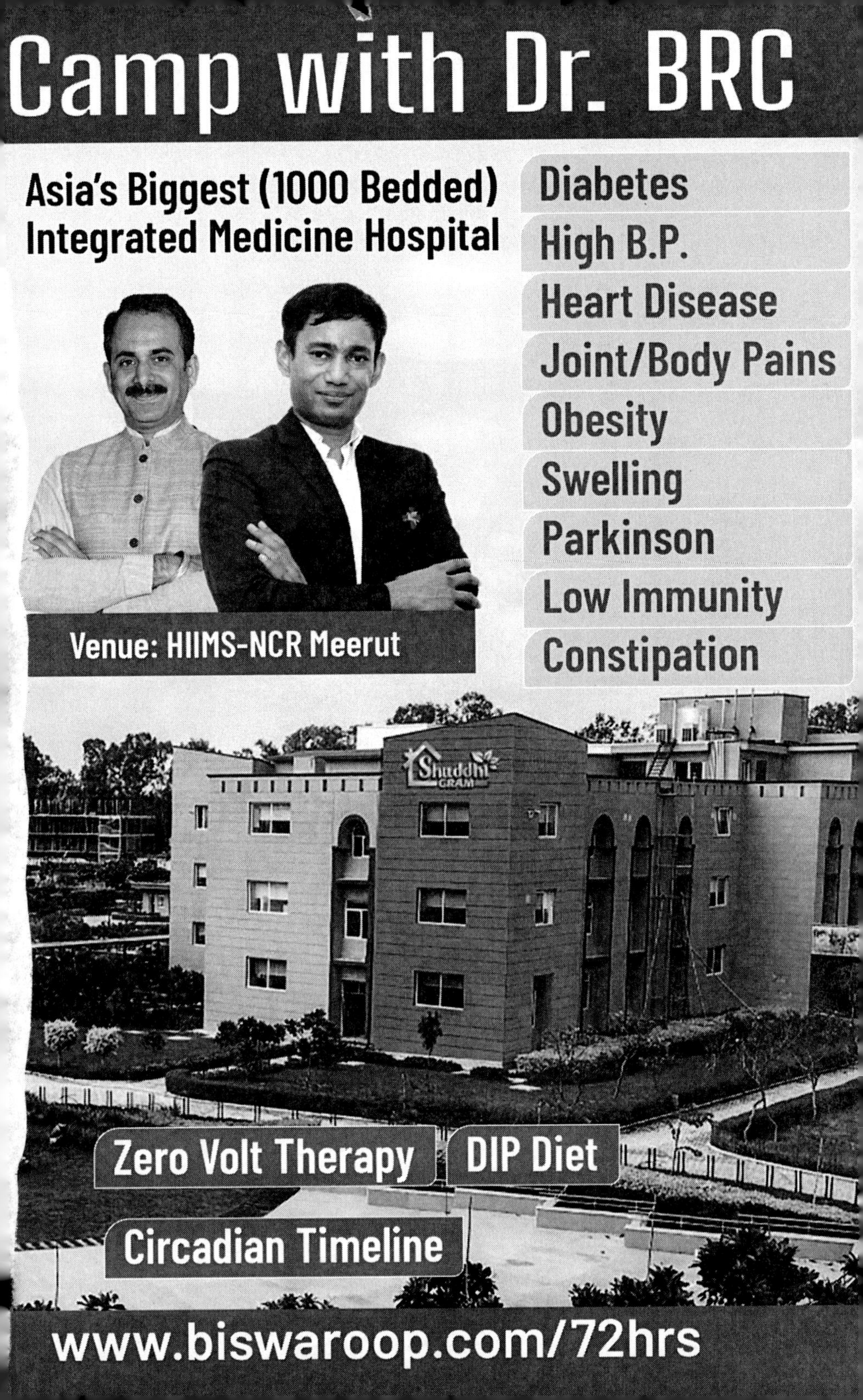
Camp with Dr. BRC
Asia's Biggest (1000 Bedded)
Integrated Medicine Hospital
Diabetes
High B.P.
Heart Disease
Joint/Body Pains
Obesity
Swelling
Parkinson
Low Immunity
Constipation
Venue: HIIMS-NCR Meerut
Shuddhi GRAM
Zero Volt Therapy
DIP Diet
Circadian Timeline
www.biswaroop.com/72hrs